PLAYING LIFE

KATHLEEN M WADDINGTON

MIND FULL READS

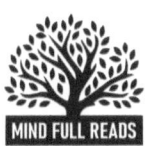

Playing Life © 2024 Kathleen M Waddington

All Rights Reserved. No part of this book may be reproduced in any form or by any electronic or mechanical means including information storage and retrieval systems, without permission in writing from the author. The only exception is by a reviewer, who may quote short excerpts in a review.

This book is a work of non-fiction. This publication is designed to provide accurate and authoritative information in regards to the subject matter covered. It is sold with the understanding that neither the author nor the publisher is engaged in rendering legal, investment, accounting, or other professional services.

Printed in Australia

Cover by Kit Cronk Studio @kitstercronk

Internal design by Book Burrow www.bookburrow.com.au

First printing: December 2024

Paperback ISBN 978-1-7637-7070-6

eBook ISBN 978-1-7637-7071-3

Distributed by Lightning Source

www.kathleenmwaddington.com

 A catalogue record for this work is available from the National Library of Australia

Also by Kathleen M. Waddington

Parent and Child - The Two Person Family

About the Author

Kathleen M Waddington is a single parent to one adult child and resides in Melbourne. She has always been interested in helping people which attracted her to the healthcare profession. She currently works as a nurse, midwife and hypnobirthing practitioner. In recent years she became aware of how expressive writing could help others in their life journey and her first book, *Parent and Child - The Two Person Family,* was published to guide and inspire other single parents. Much of the content of this book was applicable to a wider audience, so with a combination of research, her expertise in health and through her own life experiences she created a book on the analysis of life. She is now in her sixth decade as a life student. Waddington has also published articles in Pathways to Family Wellness and Bub Hub magazines.
Visit www.kathleenmwaddington.com for more information.

To you, dear reader, with whom I play life alongside; past, present and future.

CONTENTS

1   PREFACE
3   INTRODUCTION

PART ONE
Navigating the Game Board
11   LIFE'S MISHAPS
14   HUMBLE BEGINNINGS
19   THE STAGES OF LIFE
30   BODY LANGUAGE

PART TWO
Keeping Up the Pace
45   TECHNOLOGY
58   EXPECTATIONS
66   PERFECTION
74   COMPARISONS

PART THREE
Importance of Time
83   LIVING IN THE PRESENT

93	A WASTE OF TIME
98	SPONTANEOUS QUIET TIME
104	THE POWER OF NO
112	EXCUSITIS

PART FOUR
Choice Cards

123	WHAT IS GOOD ENOUGH
130	COMPONENTS OF HEALTH
153	DEALING WITH STRESS
169	HAPPINESS

PART FIVE
Surprise Cards

191	LIFE HAPPENS
195	DEALING WITH WHAT LIFE SERVES UP
203	ILLNESS
212	AMBIGUOUS LOSS
221	DEATH
242	CONCLUSION

PREFACE

I thought it would be fun to write a book about life, simulating it to a game, as all life's participants have to diligently choose their moves. I don't profess to understand the meaning of life. It is different for everyone with many similarities and uniqueness. What I have acknowledged is, all humans tend to aspire to achieve the same goals, those being: to live purposeful lives, form meaningful relationships and enjoy their time allocated on earth.

Life on earth is full of lessons and they are presented to us in many forms. Some of these lessons are obvious and some are subliminal, only evident well after an event has passed. Some lessons involve risk taking and others appear in unfortunate circumstances. Lessons are gifts in life, which continue to re-emerge until they are consolidated into knowledge. Once the message is received from the lesson, we can proceed through life with a better understanding of ourselves, others and the world around us.

I wrote this book with the intention of covering topics relevant to all parts of life. These include unexpected events and delicate subjects that are sometimes difficult to address. Life is surprising, it's all part of the game. There's no immunity from hardships and losses. We work out our moves as we go along. Nothing can be predicted. We stumble, fall and make mistakes. We also get up, equipped with a newfound wisdom, resilience and strength to power forward.

Like anyone else, I am just a student of life; some lessons learned and many more to go. So far, in my sixth decade, I have worked out that life runs better on a cup half full. To consider it half empty only erects barricades in an already challenging maze. What I have learned in my journey, my profession and my time here on earth, is something I can share with others, with the intent of providing something relatable for readers to ponder or have a little chuckle over.

I have always had a firm belief that life is what you make it. We can narrow our vision, especially when life presents us with difficult challenges, or we can take the plunge with a preparedness to take risks. This book is intended to attract players to a table of abundant cards.

INTRODUCTION

This game of life is challenging, intricate, fun and exciting. Throughout it, you are guaranteed to experience tears and laughter, pain and joy. As the dice rolls, there will be moments of surprise, pop-up opportunities and a selection of chance cards.

There are many pawns to contend with on the gaming board; some of which you will have close interactions with, others who will fleetingly pass you by and a few who will stick closely by your side throughout the entire game.

As you work around the board, there will be snakes you slip down and ladders you climb. All players will take turns, sometimes being able to contemplate their next move and other times having to leave it up to chance.

The game begins as soon as you are able to play it. When you first enter the game of life, there will be people who are quite experienced on the game board to guide you. First, they will roll the dice for you, then guide you in rolling the dice for yourself, before completely releasing you into the game. Once on your own, you will have begun to develop the skills to be able to play solo and learn new moves along the way. There are many challenges throughout the game and you will continue to become more skilled each time you work through these.

You enter the game not knowing what to expect or how long you will be playing and, at any stage, the game can spontaneously change tact. The rules you were following can become obsolete as the game you thought you were playing, suddenly turns into something completely different. What appeared to be simple could unexpectedly become complex, changing the whole dynamics of the game, where the strategies you had worked out so meticulously need to be ditched and new ones created.

Gamers may go out on a limb, taking risks and making mistakes, in which they may be penalised with a go to jail card or regress to the start of the game again, where they will begin over, equipped with newfound knowledge and expertise.

It is the same game, yet different for everyone in it. There will be times when each player will get stuck on challenges and take a while to advance forward and other times when challenges will be easy to navigate. These can be random and unpredictable for each individual.

Each player has a mission in the game, which isn't always evident to begin with and so lessons are learned as players progress around the board. These lessons are selective to each individual to enable them to progress through the varying levels of the game. Some of these lessons take several rolls of sixes or double ups.

It may appear that others in the game are more privileged than you, as they always climb the ladders and get the best chance cards, but it is merely an illusion as you won't always be at the same level throughout the game's entirety. So, it would be impossible for you to make judgement on how another person fares.

It is easy to compare your position with others on the game

board. However, the game is designed to be played according to the uniqueness of each individual and so challenges cannot be the exact same for everyone.

Each person plays according to the abilities they have acquired and these abilities are determined by: their guides, their intuition, their previous experience and time spent in the game.

There are abundant opportunity cards available to each and every player. These usually appear when one has developed an understanding of the game's complexities. During the game, the opportunity cards selected will have a bearing on one's position in the game. Some of the cards chosen may enable one to select moves posing an advantage, however, care must be taken in the timing of the selection of these cards as well as how they are interpreted so as not to cause a handicap.

It may be possible for you to anticipate where the game might be heading and what obstacles you might be up against, however, all cards are shuffled and placed face down so nothing is a certainty.

Parts of the game don't require much thought; you simply roll the dice and take your turn. Other parts require well thought out strategies where every decision made has an impact on the rest of the game.

There will be times when you feel stuck, preventing you from advancing in the game as unexpected barriers crop up. You can sit in these areas for a while to rest and reflect. This contemplation will give you renewed clarity which enables the ability to move forward. These forward moves will require constructive thinking or calculated risks to get you through to the next level.

Some components of the game will be locked until you

develop the necessary skills to unlock them. This can take patience and time. Becoming skilled at the game requires experience, some of which you will acquire along the way with practice and some of which you will have to work hard to achieve.

To perform at your best, particularly as you are unsure of the simplicity or complexity of the game, it is best to keep in top shape, both physically and mentally, at all times. Failing to do so will affect your abilities and required skills and it may even shorten your time in the game.

You may find ways of cheating, however, in doing so, you take the risk of it being to the detriment of yourself or some other player. The temptation is enticing as you could initially advance more quickly around the board, skipping difficult tasks and prematurely unlocking components that otherwise require mastery of the game. Caution needs to be taken though, as some methods of cheating can cause premature dismissal.

There is no way to predict what will happen next in the game, however, if you follow the rules carefully and take note of how you performed in previous levels, you will be at an advantage of being able to complete new tasks and challenges as they arise.

We all have a set time in the game. This time isn't revealed to us, however, we assume that we will get a substantial opportunity to play out all components. When we exit the game, it will still exist for those remaining on the board as well as for new members who are just entering. When the finish line is reached, there are no more rolls of the dice, no chance of going backwards. All we have in the end is a reflection on the way in which we played.

We will be memorable participants to those with whom

we have played alongside and, depending on the methods by which we played, some of us will have made a lasting impact on many other players we have not necessarily had close relations with or even met in the game.

Playing the game to the best of our ability is all that is required. Scooping up as many opportunity cards, taking calculated risks and exercising courage will positively influence our time in the game. The way we play can also impact other game members, even well after our departure. The knowledge gained from our progress and setbacks can be shared with others, leaving them tools to assist them in forward movement through the various levels. You may have worked hard at obtaining a golden key, unlocking components others haven't and, as a departing gift you can leave this on the game board. This will be your legacy.

PART ONE

● ● ● ●

Navigating the Game Board

LIFE'S MISHAPS

Here we are, in a life that isn't perfect (damn it!) and yet, we maintain high expectations that it mostly should be or, at least, most of the time things should go our way as we planned. No matter how hard we strive for perfection, there's really no such thing. Huh! Deep down we already know this but it's no real consolation when things go belly up.

It seems that we sometimes have control over life events and at other times we don't. We make plans, map out our life as we believe it should occur. We write our own story, so to speak, expecting every chapter to reveal everything exactly as we have planned. I's dotted; t's crossed – all of it. Yet despite our best efforts, when we review past events, looking back through the chapters we have already lived in our personal life story, we find flaws.

Throughout our lives, there will be things that don't go our way, expected events that don't happen, unexpected events that do happen, and plans that we need to put on hold or cancel altogether. On reflection, we may feel disappointed in life, upset, even angry that it didn't pan out the way we believe it should have. We wonder what we did wrong, questioning why our path veered off course. After all, it had no right to take us on an unexpected road when we had pre-set our life navigation very specifically! And even though those predetermined settings were accurately entered, something or someone upset the course by sneaking in to make changes. So, we cop it on the chin, accepting that life has its twists and turns.

We all encounter things in our lives that weren't a part of our expectations. Events happen. Sometimes because of the choices we make and other times, resulting from circumstances out of our control. We are quick to blame ourselves for our misfortunes and misdemeanours, as we are intellectual beings capable of organising our lives and our deepest desire is to have control. We want to have a tidy life and when it becomes messy, we feel as though we have failed in some way or that life has been unfair to us.

What can we do when life doesn't go our way, when we are dealt the dud cards? When life becomes topsy-turvy, we need to draw out our big guns – not to shoot it down or turn them on ourselves, but to give us the confidence that we have the ammunition to deal with whatever life throws at us.

We can choose the ammunition we purchase. We are not at the mercy of life. We are human and, as such, we are imperfect beings. We make mistakes. We have misconceptions and fears. This is all normal; it is part of our makeup. We are also capable of: making good decisions, accumulating wisdom and eliminating situations that cause trepidation.

There are events that are out of our control: death, disease, earthquakes, tsunamis and other life catastrophes. These events require the best ammunition our minds can master. As difficult as these challenges are, we can surprisingly move through them with the advantage of gaining something positive from them. Our mindset will determine our behaviour and how we handle adversity. So, let's load up with rounds of superior ammunition – the best our minds can custom design.

We live in anticipation of something exciting or surprising happening, constantly seeking a richer more deeply satisfying life. We need to meet our most basic needs of food, water, shelter and sleep to survive. Beyond this, we need to feel connected to others and fulfil desires that propel us forward, giving us purpose. True satisfaction may be derived from: relationships we form, career pathways and projects we undertake, tributes we make and legacies we create.

There's no life manual on how best to live it. Each one of us is born with a particular disposition and placed in a specific environment. We have no conscious memory of deciding in which country to be born, who our parents will be and even if they will be involved in our upbringing. Who knows, maybe we did get to choose our circumstances preceding birth, but once born, we have no recollection of any such choices. Our life situations are all unique and the environment in which we begin our formative years will have an impact on the way in which we develop, influencing our thoughts, actions and belief systems, from which our behaviours originate. These behaviours have a huge effect on our successes in life. However, it is not only the formative years that mould us. Life continues on and we evolve as new experiences are presented to us, forever learning and adding new dimensions to our being.

Life isn't perfect. There are times we feel we are on a winning streak and times when we feel defeated; times that we feel elated and times we feel disheartened. We can't win or lose life's game; we can only equip ourselves to live the best life possible.

HUMBLE BEGINNINGS

We are born. Quick check – yes, all there. Phew, no major deformities. We have made it through the passage of pregnancy unscathed or, at least, to our knowledge not noticeably so.

Have you heard of the saying, 'He was born with a silver spoon in his mouth'? This tends to mean you are born with privileges, usually along the lines of wealth and social status. You may not have to work as hard as others might to acquire riches or prestige, as you have been gifted them. There is no need to prove your worth or reputation as these have already been programmed into your being.

Well, what happens if you were born with a brass spoon, no spoon or just plain dirt in your mouth? We have no control over what family or country we are born into and so we may start off at a disadvantage. This disadvantage may even begin before we are released into the world. Birth, in itself, can be an obstacle course and we may come through it battered and bruised. Thankfully, nowadays with improved technology and fetal surveillance, there is close observation throughout the process, but that really depends on which destination the gods send your package.

There is a better breed of baby storks in the western world than in the eastern and third world countries. In the developed affluent world, care begins even before becoming pregnant. There are support vitamins you can purchase prior to becoming pregnant. There are also fertility clinics and IVF options to assist in achieving a pregnancy. Once pregnant, the support continues with prenatal care, including numerous blood tests, ultrasounds and continuous surveillance on fetal development and wellbeing. In the less affluent world, support structures are reduced due to limited resources. Any which way we arrive, we begin our life's journey naked in every sense of the word. We are only equipped with our cuteness, totally reliant on the long-term occupants of the world.

As long as we are alive, we have the opportunity of making the best of our world with the assets we have and the choices we make. Some of us may never acquire riches or have the opportunity to acquire the best education. This doesn't mean you can't still live a long, happy life. Look at people who live in third world countries; it is enlightening to see how happy they can be, despite their scant possessions and opportunities in life. Maybe it's because they don't experience the stress that often accompanies the pretentious world of working hard to acquire riches thought to be necessary for a "good life". In fact, striving to keep up leaves little time for the essential things in life that we need and crave: rest and relaxation, time spent with loved ones, exercise and enjoying the simple things. It is so easy to get caught up in the stressors in an attempt to get ahead in life that we forget to slow down and simply enjoy living.

The less complicated our world is, the more time we have to appreciate what we have at hand. Constantly negotiating the fast lane in life obliterates the present moment.

We all have disappointments of some kind or another, despite our status in life. You may have wished: to have been born in a different country, to be born to a different family, for a family of your own, to have two parents instead of one, have at least one parent, siblings if you don't have or rather have been an only child. You may have inherited curly hair but you wanted straight, fair freckled skin when you would have preferred a flawless olive complexion. There are many things that may cause disappointment in your life. Conversely, there are many things to be grateful for.

Gratitude is an appreciation of the good things in life. It doesn't require that you have come from the best gene stock, that you have to own something big, have accumulated a collection of trophies or awards, graduated from college or sought out a prestigious job. Gratitude comes from an appreciation of what you have and what you can give out to the world. The simplest things in life can cut it.

To accumulate more gratitude in our lives, we need to be open to the present. Our minds are often in travel mode, randomly switching from past to future and rarely staying too long in the present. It is only when we are truly in the present that we become aware of our being and everything around us. It is then we are privy to a kaleidoscopic view of what we have to be thankful for.

Being thankful is an essential part of happiness. If we could stop our minds dwelling on past events and what might happen in the future and just park for a while in the realm of now, then we diminish our worries and concerns that stem from our mind travel. With a freer more open mind, we become receptive to our consciousness, erecting our antennae to bring in more signals from our surrounds.

Learning to switch off can take practice and patience. Liken the mind to an iceberg; the conscious part sits above the water and the subconscious part is what lies below the surface. Within the subconscious mind lie all your thoughts, feelings, conditioning and memories and it is continually sorting through stuff. The busyness of the downstairs department can distract what is happening upstairs and so the conscious mind battles to be fully aware in the present moment.

To be able to experience everything in our immediate surrounds, we need to switch off or, at the very least, turn down our internal dialogue. It is only then that the world really opens up and we can perceive everything in it. Not only are we more attentive to the sights, smells and sounds around us, we are also perceptive to all its dimensions. It is in this state we are able to become more connected to our feelings, which opens the door to gratitude.

To be grateful means being aware of what is present and abundant, of all that is good in life from the simplest of things to the grandest. It's a feeling that comes when you notice and appreciate the moments in life. We can easily miss life as it happens because we are not in tune with it. Instead, we are busy in our heads, distracted from fully engaging in the now. When we quieten our mind, we open up all our senses and become receptive to the richness of the world.

As a child, all that exists in life is the moment. There is no concept of past or present dragging your thoughts around and dulling your senses. What you have is the presence of now and so you enjoy and absorb every part of it. As we move through the passage of life, we can become desensitised to the enjoyment of the moment, as many of our experiences are repeated and our minds become busier, downloading an influx of data that requires "thinking time" to sort through.

Think about when you were a child and how you viewed

the world. Your mind was open to every new experience and you delighted in all your new discoveries as the world gradually revealed its magic. There was no sense of time, no hurrying through events. Why not practice seeing life through a child's eyes? You may notice when you play with a child and are really engaged with them, the yesterdays and tomorrows, that so often overshadow your thoughts, fall away from your consciousness and you may surprise yourself at how liberated you feel in the moment.

As we move out of childhood into adulthood, the world becomes frightfully busy. There are adult responsibilities to deal with and expanding relationships that require a good portion of our energy. Toys have given way to an accumulation of possessions and these possessions require maintenance. More time required. The once empty, only live in the moment, headspace fills with thoughts we pluck out of the past and plans we make for the future. It takes controlled effort to free up some space to be able to connect to the present. There are times we are so involved with all that we have to achieve and all that needs to be done, we frighten ourselves into realising we are not really living in the present. The moment we are supposed to be in, is all too often obscured by the cloud of our thoughts.

It is so easy to abandon the simple pleasures in life when you become overwhelmed with responsibilities and concerns, much of which stems from: other people's demands, work expectations, family commitments and advancing technology. Adjusting priorities, learning to take care of yourself, part of which may involve setting up boundaries, can free up time to spend on what's really important to you in this, your life.

THE STAGES OF LIFE

Our lives span out over a small collection of decades. Let's say that if we live a full, healthy life, we may see through 10 decades. Right now, in our lifetime, there are people in the early decades, some in the middle and some living their last few. Wherever we are on the decade scale, we are all mingled together over a relatively short period of time spanning 100 years, give or take. Given the thousands of years of humanity that have preceded us and those thousands ahead of our existence, we are collectively close in age. In perspective, we are all living within the same era at this point in time. Depending on how many decades we get to live, we will experience significant changes throughout our individual lifetime.

Let's take a look at life's stages:

Infancy/Childhood – You are completely reliant on your caregivers. You thrive if your basic needs are met including an adequate dose of love. You are a new bud awaiting bloom: delicate, precious and at the mercy of the hand that nurtures you. Your sole occupation is absorbing everything in the newness of your world, constantly feeding your brain volumes of information as it undergoes rapid development, multiplying neurons a thousandfold. There is no comprehension of past or present as you live totally in the moment; unaware of the continuum of time, completely involved in anything that stimulates your senses. Your being is the main focus of your world. Little do you understand of anyone else occupying the planet. The most serious threat in your life would be falling over, stranger danger or becoming lost.

Adults are your lifeline. They dress you, feed you, take you places, entertain you and put you to bed. Incapable of making decisions for yourself, they are all made for you. You have no capacity to think beyond the moment. You are unable to recall the events of yesterday and you don't anticipate that there will be another day that follows the one you are in. At this stage, your subconscious mind is in its early development and so doesn't interrupt your thoughts pulling you away from the present as it does in later stages of your life.

You don't care about worldly possessions as they are not relevant to your lifestyle. You view adults as being the lucky ones. You are told that your life is easy but you think otherwise, as you are constricted by those in authority. You eagerly wait to grow up, so you can live by your own rules and have your own money to spend on infinite amounts of candy and toys.

Youth – Your skin is taut; you have boundless energy and a spring in your step. You are innocent, still having so much to learn about life. Your decision making is purely emotional as rational thought hasn't yet fully matured. You feel invincible, you are experimenting, you take risks. Life is for living and you figure that you have plenty of it in front of you. You may push boundaries as you are keen to discover everything that life has to offer. You soak in each new experience in awe, crisp in its newness.

There are many stumbling blocks as you establish who you are and where you want to go but these are just lessons learned and you proceed to the next chapter enthusiastically. You discover limitations through your own personal experience. Those ahead of you in life's game may throw down some stepping stones to assist you through the levels but you mostly prefer to devise your own moves. Even if there are things you want to change, you are at this stage looking your best. You can only travel forward in life and, in comparison to those who are further along the road, you are acutely aware that you are at your physical peak. You take advantage of this, feeling somewhat superior to those much older than you. Many of your plans are short term as much of life is still ahead of you and you eagerly look forward to the future as there are so many experiences yet to be had.

Adulthood – You are finally where you longed to be. Grownup. Independent. You had been counting the years wishing to be older so you could take full hold of the reins. Now the reins are in your hands! Finally, you are free to make your own decisions. Yes, you may have parents in the background trying to influence these decisions, as in their eyes you are still their child and it is difficult for them to identify a time when you hatched into an adult. This can make you feel supported or hindered, or a bit of both sometimes.

For the first time in your life, you think beyond the present and begin to make long term plans. You have freedom. You tackle new challenges on the horizon with enthusiasm as you get to exercise your newfound capabilities. At this point, you no longer want to fast forward the years. In fact, you would quite happily repeat a few birthdays with 25 candles. As you experience the responsibilities that come with adulthood, you comprehend the meaning of a simple life in childhood.

Middle Aged – You have gathered a repertoire of

experiences that have laid down your foundations. At this stage, you have reached a level of maturity and self-satisfaction to feel more comfortable in life. You may not have as many new experiences as those that are repeated, through which develops expertise. Through your many experiences you can now decipher what is and who is or isn't important to you. Your maturity helps you to prioritise; evaluate what you are good at and who benefits you in life.

You begin to step back from worldly responsibilities to reflect on the deeper meaning of life. You begin to make more time for yourself, selective of the people you want to remain in your life. You may go through a period of grieving your younger years. You once looked forward to those years with an anticipation of all that lay ahead of you and now you have reached them. You sometimes find yourself catching your thoughts regarding what you will do when you "grow up" as your mind sometimes tricks you into believing that you still have that time ahead. The beginning of grey hairs and fine lines confirm that you have overtaken youth and you may feel somewhat resentful that you cannot rewind time. Products that camouflage the beginnings of the ageing process are added to your shopping list.

Getting Older – It finally dawns on you that "life is short". You are the same person on the inside, yet your outside wrapping has changed. You frighten yourself sometimes when you look in the mirror. Your eyes see the same world and you feel the same as you did as a younger version of yourself, so how is it that the image portrays a different picture of you? You had forgotten just how fast the last 20 years flew by and now you have to accept that the body has been subject to the gravitational pull, disfiguring the great assets you once had.

Just when you feel comfortable in your skin, you notice that it has become a rather loose fit than it once was and remedies that bring back some youthfulness, spark your interest. It would be nice to tighten up your features even if it's just a smidgen. If a person thinks that you are younger than your true age you take it as a compliment. You begin to spend time reflecting, recalling treasured memories you carefully filed throughout the chapters of your life. This is a time of pausing, of taking time to reminisce through the photo album of your life. Life becomes simpler as you step away from the flurry of building a career and/or raising a family. If you are still working, you have well and truly established your skills and don't need to prove these to anyone. You may have silenced the wolf whistler when taking a stroll through the streets but on hearing one, you glance back at an awkward youth, now a fond memory of a time when you were once young and still establishing your identity.

Old Age – Looking in the mirror, there's no denying it. It really is you living in a body that your grandparent used to live in. You expected to grow older but that was always in the distant future and now the truth hits you like a ton of bricks – the body just doesn't last forever and that once distant future now becomes your present.

The pedestrian crossing you once sprinted across becomes an obstacle course and you desperately hope your slow shuffle gets you to the other side before the lights change. Even though you have aged, your inner being still feels the same and you forget how you may appear to others. Standing in line at a counter, when it's your turn to be served, you may find that the person on the other side has slowed and raised their voice at the same time, automatically expecting that you are hearing impaired, accompanied by a possibility of dementia.

This is amusing to you as it affirms a young person's perspective of old age. One it seemed you had not too long ago. You are in the senior citizen category. *How could this be?* you wonder, when in your mind you are still young. You have lived through many decades and have the advantage of knowing many worlds. You have scored many achievements of which to be proud, despite whether they are displayed as trophies or modestly kept under wraps. Even though you may have slowed down, you are wise with many life stories to share. When you were once a kid, you envisioned one day being old or else you would die young. So here you are, old age achieved!

Each stage of life is equally significant in the human life cycle. There are unique tasks presented in each given stage, which once completed, allows us a sense of competence and achievement. As a human race, we can all benefit from the gifts that each stage delivers.

Before birth, before a new life even enters the world, there is an excited anticipation of hope. Hope of what this new being will bring into the world. So, even before you are known, you ignite an interest in those expecting your arrival. There is a celebration surrounding birth as a person is welcomed into life and then again at death, to commemorate the journey one has completed.

Infancy and childhood bring joy, a sense of achievement and satisfaction to parents and other caregivers as they become instrumental in moulding a person's development. As a child learns from an adult, so too, does the adult learn from a child. Children can enlighten the seriousness of the world that an adult becomes accustomed to. There is some reprieve in being able to revisit your own childhood through child's play when you are fully grown.

The teen and young adult are still maturing and incapable of making wise decisions, hence they are reliant on those who have the acquired level of maturity to help them make good decisions. In return, the older person may benefit from the young by means of exchanging the most newly acquired knowledge, particularly in technology. Is there a person under the age of 30 who isn't a computer guru?

As the adult matures and becomes one of the senior members of society, roles may reverse with the younger members becoming more active in caring roles. This assistance can benefit the senior member on all levels: physically, mentally and spiritually, as it validates their worth. Senior citizens usually have more time on their hands, having completed their working career and raising families. They no longer live in the rush hour and so are able to savour life.

Loneliness may creep in, as well as a sense of not belonging, but that can be quashed by becoming involved in voluntary work or having free time to mentor the young. The benefits are twofold: the youth get to receive attention and mentoring they may otherwise lack and the elder gets to practice cognitive skills and serve a new purpose to fulfil their life. Having already lived many chapters, there is an abundance of acquired wisdom through life experiences that can be imparted onto others and readily so as the elders come back to living in the "now", not bogged down by the incessant chatter that so often occupies the mind of their younger counterpart.

We mostly live in a society that celebrates youth. We tend to hide our age after our first quarter century. Children are quick to tell you their age, eagerly wishing to be older.

'I'm nine and a half.'

No one tells you they are 65 and a half. In fact, it's not acceptable to ask anyone over 30 their age. We like to pretend that we are younger than what we really are when we reach our middle years, as if ageing is something we should try to hide or be ashamed of. Comments such as: I didn't think you were that old/you look good for your age/over the hill/not too many years left and birthday cards with sarcastic slogans about getting older, can make us want to retreat back into our shell.

We should be made to feel proud of our advancing age, of all of our achievements and accumulated knowledge. It is only through ageing that we develop many skills and abilities, as they have been practised over and over again, putting us at an advantage over the younger population. This should give us confidence and respect and make us popular as we become the "go to" people of the world. Everyone is now privy to an abundance of information at the press of their fingers, but wisdom can only be dispersed on consulting with someone who has obtained many life experiences and who better than a mature aged citizen?

What is the reason, when we grow old, that all body functions slow down? If we maintained our youthful appearance, we could perhaps forget our age and kid ourselves into thinking we are invincible. If we live into our eighth, ninth or tenth decade then we have been privileged to have experienced much of life and it is time to relax and reflect. A time to be proud of our achievements and the many chapters of life we have been a part of. As difficult as it may be to accept the changes that are occurring in our bodies, we should wear them graciously, knowing we have made it to the last chapters, proud of all that we have achieved in the previous chapters.

On reflection, we may have some regrets, wishing life may have panned out somewhat differently for us. We may even compare our lives with others who seem to have had a smoother run. We can't live in another's shoes and what appears to be what we may think is a better life, is only in our limited perception. Every one of us in this human race has challenges, different they may be, but better or worse, we are incapable of judging. Life will have its "ups and downs" for everyone. No one can purchase an immunity card. The difficulties we encounter create valuable lessons, which, once worked through, open up new opportunities and enrich our lives, no matter what our age.

Yearning for our youth can be a part of missing the excitement of experiences we have become accustomed to. When experiences are repeated over and over as they are with time, familiarity makes us somewhat more insensitive to their enjoyment. We remember the elation, delight and surprise of when we first encounter a particular experience and we crave to feel that again, however, it is never quite the same when we repeat the same experience. It is easy to become complacent with what is familiar to us and so we live life doing the same of many things. Despite infinite unique experiences available to us, we mostly stick to what we know.

Reinvigorating your life may mean stepping out of your comfort zone or simply making a conscious effort (which may entail locking in a date) to do something new, something different, something that creates that first time thrill and another memory to lock away.

As we grow older, our peripheral vision narrows, so much of our experiences have already been snapshot and filed into compartments of the mind. So, things we repeatedly see, touch and smell don't make as an impression as they once did. Instead of enjoying a panoramic view of the world, we tend to narrow our focus, limiting our experiences. A way of overcoming this is to be mindful of engaging all senses in the present moment. This will widen your vision, taking you back to viewing life through the eyes of a child, before mind chatter and clutter distorted your perception.

We enter life then depart from it. We all have a road to travel. On this road, we meet others, some of whom we connect with and others with whom we don't, necessarily. Sometimes we help people in their journey and sometimes they help us. There are people in our lives that we will form close bonds with and others with whom we won't. Intuitively, we select those who benefit us in life. Some of these people come and go throughout our lifetime and others are with us from beginning to end. Sometimes, we may wonder why we have people in our lives that we don't particularly connect with. These relationships may include family members, work colleagues and acquaintances. Despite not forming particularly strong bonds with these people, they provide us with valuable lessons necessary for personal growth. Regardless of who we travel alongside during life's journey, there are many people of varying ages who are instrumental in many of our ventures.

Whatever your stage in life, you have always and will always be you, regardless of the physical form you occupy at this present moment. You were once you in a baby body, as you were in a child's body and it is the same you, residing in an adolescent or adult frame. You pass through the stages of life never exclusively remaining in the one form and never exempt from changing physical forms. What is important to remember is your essence is the same, as you travel through these evolving forms.

BODY LANGUAGE

At the beginning of life, before language is learned, a baby's only form of communication is through body language. This gives the caregiver important cues on what a baby needs and how he or she is feeling. To pick up on these cues, adults need to pay close attention to different kinds of crying, facial expressions and body movements. As the baby develops, vowel sounds begin, eventually leading to verbal communication.

Even when language is mastered, a huge part of what we are communicating comes from body signals: our posture, stance, gestures and facial expressions. So many cues can be picked up in non-verbal language, on both conscious and subconscious levels, that it bears more credibility than spoken words. It reveals the truth of what we are really conveying.

Communication is a part of our being. When we think about communication, we concentrate on the spoken or written language. We are mostly in control of how our speech is received by our choice of words, the tone of our voice and the way in which we construct our sentences. However, the body doesn't have the same composure and will deliver cues that either cement or unravel what has been said. Although we speak on a conscious level, we are not always aware we are also communicating in a non-verbal way which is easily recognised and decoded by our audience.

Instead of one universal language in the world, there are thousands of different languages spread across the globe. Migration and education have enabled people to learn and speak more than one language, however, there remains a diversity of languages throughout the world. No one really knows how language developed differently. It is thought to be due to distance and time. As people migrated away from one another, dialects changed, eventually forming new versions of language.

There are multilingual people, however, there are up to 7,000 different languages globally and it would be impossible to learn them all. At some stage in our lives, we are bound to face a language barrier. As we struggle to find suitable words, we often give over to body language universally communicated. We can even attempt our own designed sign language to help transmit information. Irrespective of understanding the words exchanged, we can usually manage some sort of understanding and connection through body expressions. After all, in the very beginning of human life, this is all people had until words were invented.

Body language can be beautifully captured in early film making. In the late 1800s, the very first movies were created without dialogue before the means of synchronising sound. Apart from the use of title cards, the story was conveyed using exaggerated body language. The heavy makeup, used to suit poor film lighting at the time, also served to accentuate facial expressions. The music that accompanied the silent film, not only camouflaged the noise of the projector, it added to the over-dramatisation of the role playing.

The way you walk, the manner in which you speak, the expression on your face, even the space you occupy, sends out messages to the world about how you are feeling and the way in which you perceive yourself. Others pick up on the cues you portray and subconsciously make a judgement. The words you speak are meaningless, if the tone of your voice or body language sends out a different message. It doesn't matter if you choose your words carefully, nonverbal signals carry more impact and you can be easily read on a subliminal level. When nonverbal signals don't match the words spoken, what is being communicated becomes confusing to the recipient. The power of body language will overrule and these nonverbal cues go on to become the foundation of hunches and gut feelings from which an impression is formed.

Our facial expressions often mask what we are really feeling. We discipline our faces to not reveal any unsavoury emotions. What we are feeling on the inside is often camouflaged by the mask we wear. Smiling is perceived as a social nicety and, despite our emotional status, we can fake smile in politeness at strangers, acquaintances, colleagues, friends and family. These smiles disguise our present frame of mind. They are props enabling us to behave in a socially acceptable way, keeping others comfortable, preventing them from delving into our true feelings.

There are masks which are temporarily worn as a sign of greeting or of expressing humour. How many times do we fake smile or laugh at something we don't even find funny? A smile can cleverly conceal true emotions. It can also be worn as a gesture of an apology, an annoyance, a sign of defence or as an excuse. A smile can get us through the day, even if underneath we feel angry or frustrated. To avoid confrontation of real feelings or invasion of privacy, it can be easier to just don an appropriate mask and pretend something else. That way we can swiftly move through life's moments, bypassing the inconvenience of exposing and dealing with unwanted emotions.

When we are in proximity to others, there is an etiquette to be withheld. We automatically hold ourselves in control, lest we spill the beans on what our minds are desperately trying to conceal. If we were to lose this control, it could lead to unsavoury or embarrassing behaviour that could taint our personality and likeability.

Our masks can be removed in the confines of our own space. Take being in a car for instance. We are in a protective space where we can let down our guard completely. Encased in our metallic cocoon, there are no inhibitions as we let loose on the person that cut us off or stole our car park. Unlike a face-to-face confrontation, we have armour to shield us should we need it in the case of retaliation. We are in our own zone and free from pretence, with the added advantage of being able to flee quickly from any unwanted repercussions. We may even surprise ourselves with an explosive release of pent-up anger, as there is no mask required to keep a lid on it.

We can also reveal our emotional nakedness in the presence of family members or close friends. We know these people accept us unconditionally and so we feel safe in exposing our true selves. Other times, we may forfeit the mask, include times of illness and total dependence. There is no need to disguise our feelings as we have good reason to validate them. We surrender our wellbeing to the judgement of our carers, whom we are temporarily, or even permanently, reliant on. Precariously, we give over our masks in full trust of our carer being respectful of our most vulnerable state and hope for the best.

Some people treat others as though they don't matter, as though they are inferior or unimportant in some way. These people don't bother to camouflage anything with the use of a mask and so behave, oblivious to the feeling of or respect for another person. It may be they feel superior because of social status, race or merely on the basis of a biased opinion formed.

There are times when the mask is tightened to completely ignore someone – the beggar or crazy man in the street. We may bypass someone we know well but don't have the time or inclination to stop what we are doing to exchange pleasantries and engage in unwanted conversation. So, we pretend we didn't see them and move on. If we accidentally come face up to them, we will make up some feeble excuse.

'Oh, it is you! I'm short sighted these days/wasn't wearing my glasses.'

Who knows, that same person could just as well have been avoiding us for the same reasons we steered clear of them! Sometimes the busyness of life just gets in the way. It's not our intention to dismiss these people, it's just an easier option at the moment to do so. Of course, there can be an underlying feeling of uneasiness following such encounters, particularly if eyes were briefly locked in an accidental glance.

Know that there is no need to feel embarrassed or awkward as we are all culprits of the same behaviour and this is usually mutually understood by the person you avoided. Life carries on and the next meeting you have with that same person may be in a social setting, when you both have time to enjoy the engagement of pleasantries you previously desperately steered clear of. Each of you acknowledges that the last time you saw one another, or rather pretended you didn't, doesn't matter as you were wearing the mask of, 'I don't want to be noticed'. Hence, nothing needs to be said as you both share an unspoken understanding of the previous encounter.

Who of you remembers the Looney Tunes cartoon, "Ralph Wolf and Sam Sheepdog"? This animation exaggerates the different masks people wear to suit their settings. In the cartoon, the two characters begin the day by exchanging pleasantries as they clock on to their work shift. As soon as the cards are punched in, they immediately throw off their masks and adopt two different personas to characterise their working conditions. Governed by their natural instincts, they each become antagonistic toward the other, right up until the whistle blows indicating the end of their working day. Always saved by the whistle and just shy of killing one another, the masks of society spring back into place. They make their stroll home together, happily chatting and wishing each other a good night with an eagerness of meeting again in the morning as mutually respectful colleagues, before they once again turn on one another when the workday begins.

Although most of us are unlikely to go as far as the extremes of Ralph and Sam, there are two different personas we traverse between in both our professional and home lives. Depending on a person's character and their position in the workplace, these alternating personas can be markedly different, as they adapt to best suit their different situations. Amongst the basket of many, an appropriate mask is chosen to best enhance one's professional and personal success.

Like characters in a stage show, we don different costumes for different settings. Sometimes we are aware of changing our attire and sometimes the changes are only noticeable to others. Our performance in the home setting differs from the school setting, work setting or social setting. There are also notable changes in more serious settings such as doing a public speech, chairing a meeting, being an active participant in a courtroom or performing on a stage. We all adopt different personas according to the settings we find ourselves in and tailor our behaviours to best suit the situation. We can be many characters on life's stage.

Body language is often revealed in unconscious gestures, whereas we engage our thoughts before we speak. Sometimes, we may not construct our sentences too well or we may experience a slip of the tongue, however, we mostly always put thought into what we say. Our gestures are more automatic, so what we portray in our nonverbal communication is a true display of our real thoughts and intentions. Many of the signals portrayed in body language are read by others on a subliminal level and an opinion is formed. So, if body gestures mismatch what is spoken, the words may not hold merit, giving a different impression to that of what was so carefully articulated.

We may mimic others with our body language, especially when we connect and are in flow with one another. When we don't connect with another, our body language may be in total opposition. This is an automatic response that occurs on a subconscious level. Think of how you behave when you are in a social event. There are some people present that you know and really like and there could be others you would rather not give the time of day. You would naturally be showing your enjoyment or discomfort in your body language. Even though the conversation remains courteous in each of these respective encounters, it is more difficult to mask body language. True emotions can be revealed in the way we hold ourselves. When there is no connection, we could appear fidgety or easily distracted as, despite our best attempt at pleasantries, it is difficult to conceal the discomfort we feel as our mind busily formulates an escape from an unpleasant situation.

Why do we intuitively know when a person likes us or not? It is something we sense in the vibes of body language. What if we were to be truthful all of the time? As children, we observe and report things as they are.

'She shouldn't be here, she's too fat!' stated my son in a KFC restaurant.

My child, a mere seven-year-old, was left confused and bewildered when his mouth was instantly clasped shut by my own oversized adult hand with demands of, 'Shush, you can't say that!'

As we proceed to adulthood, we learn to conform to society. We must learn to disguise our true thoughts and feelings in order to protect ourselves and others from humiliation. We learn to express our positive emotions and camouflage our negative ones. And so, we create an array of masks to best suit the inhibitions that society places upon us. We replace our freedom of expression with a mask of protection.

I think we all know of people that don't have a filter. They don't contain their thoughts or emotions but rather blurt out what's on their minds, without considering the consequences. They say it as it is, with no effort to withhold anything that may be offensive, embarrassing or intimidating. Although honest, these people can be hurtful through their use of words. We all value honesty but there is a tactful way of delivering it with language. The harshness of honesty can be softened with the proper selection of words in any given situation. It may also require a particular setting or timing.

Once at a nightclub, a male acquaintance blatantly pointed out I was no oil painting. Duh...yes, I know but I had put some extra effort in my appearance before stepping out that night! *Thanks a lot,* I thought, feeling like telling him that he was a pretty ordinary specimen himself. Shocked he had the audacity, I withheld retaliation. At times we have all been subject to blunt, tactless comments. On the odd occasion we have let slip something inappropriate ourselves.

If our verbal communication was always truthful, we wouldn't rely so much on nonverbal language. Words have to be chosen carefully to not offend or conjure up negative emotions causing communication to shut down. Thus, we have to become efficient in reading the nonverbal addition of communication to understand what is truly conveyed in language.

We are able to pick up many subtle signals in body language that convey what a person is feeling, in conjunction with the words they are using. This body language will either marry or be in opposition of the selected words used. Language then becomes a collection of words, movements, facial expressions and body posture, from which we can decipher honesty and integrity. The words spoken are only a part of the equation and cannot suffice to provide the whole meaning of communication. The unspoken element of communication helps us to understand the complete message of what someone is conveying to us. Even though a person selectively crafts words to accomplish their objective, they are often unaware of how their nonverbal behaviours reveal the truth behind the words they choose.

A subliminal opinion will be formed on the nonverbal components of language giving us a "feeling" about another which denotes trust or distrust. Words alone cannot give us sufficient information to form an adequate judgement of one's character.

Body language is bypassed when we engage in phone conversation, written letters, emails and social media. We have to rely completely on tone of voice and choice of words. In a written form, punctuation marks can assist in our interpretation of the meaning and feeling behind what is said. However, without the assistance of what we read in body language, even well-structured sentences can leave us bewildered to the true meaning in the message.

Correspondence in the form of letter writing, text messaging or emails, often include a context of courtesy words or emoticons which help convey the authenticity of the message, however, they can also create an illusion. It is a medium for which a mask can easily be donned and the audience is none the wiser. Without the ability to receive nonverbal cues, a lot can be lost in translation. Does something written in all capitals indicate anger? Does a short response mean disinterest or was it just written in a hurry? Is an over-embellished text sincere? What about a delayed response? As devices are now at our fingertips, we expect the receiver to respond fairly promptly and if the delay is substantial, we are quick to fabricate reasons why. In reality, we know there could be many reasons for a delayed response as our form of communication isn't in real time, however, latency can be a recipe for misinterpretation.

Computer-mediated communication can take away the awkwardness of face-to-face communication facilitating an ease of correspondence between two parties. Online dating has become a popular means of becoming acquainted. This platform only requires verbal communication. There is no need to worry about appearance or embarrassing gestures, which may discredit first impressions. The whole person can be revealed after preliminaries are met. Once the parties have become comfortable with one another, screens can give way to real life interaction. It is then when nonverbal communication will either strengthen or weaken personal connections.

Humans are a social species who need to form connections with other people throughout life. Body language is an important tool in expressing our feelings for one another. Mirroring is a sign of being in sync with another, of feeling comfort, trust and rapport. When we feel a harmonious connection, we unconsciously reflect that by mimicking another person's posture, gestures and words. This synchronisation is so automatic we are often oblivious to it. We constantly scan the bodies of people we meet for the first time to decipher whether or not we can trust them. If they pass the test, we go on to assess their feelings towards us. If mirroring occurs in our expressive body language, it's a thumbs up. A genuine connection is made.

There are people with whom we don't want to form connections, such as those we don't like or strangers and so we would naturally avoid mimicking them in any way. Silently, we would convey an emotional distance.

We may withhold our tongues in an attempt to avoid disclosure but body language can't lie. Even the masks worn can be obvious to others, particularly when we are acutely aware that these are the norm of society. We subconsciously accept the mask even when we know it is a shield erected to protect the wearer from undesirable behaviour or consequences.

There is an etiquette of space we keep to not impose

or make another person feel uncomfortable. We may steal a glance at a stranger but won't hold the gaze too long in case we are caught. If we were caught, we would quickly divert our eyes away and pretend we weren't really staring. We would naturally space ourselves a few feet from another unknown person in a public place unless that place was crowded. Once we gain familiarity with a person, we may step a little closer and the gap narrows the more intimate we become. We may start off as strangers in a setting such as at a party or conference and within a few short hours we have become well acquainted. The masks we had erected at the beginning of the event are slowly disrobed, as we begin to feel more comfortable with people with whom we have found familiar ground.

Body language is a necessary tool we use throughout our entire lifetime. Some of it is innately automatic and some of it is learned through conditioning. Although it mostly happens unawares, before you can put thought into it, you can learn to observe and control body language to your advantage.

PART TWO

Keeping Up the Pace

TECHNOLOGY

The existence of a simple life once known to our ancestors as hunters and gatherers has been steadily replaced by the complexities of an expanding world over centuries and decades. To survive in the modern world, we have to progress lest we fall behind.

Digital technologies have bled into our lifestyles and culture, affecting our behaviour and thinking patterns. These patterns have been altered by a new focus, that of a virtual reality, where we can be submerged in a digital world far removed from our three-dimensional existence. Digital screens are everywhere in our world, many of which have a tantalising effect on the mind, drawing it away from real time activities and into a simulated world of virtual reality. Screen time makes up a large chunk of today's leisure activities.

Modern technology has accelerated interconnections, enhanced travel and medical revolution and has altered the way of communication. The internet has revolutionised the way we communicate with each other. There are many options available to suit both personal and professional forms of communication. Letters and postcards have become extinct and you no longer need to leave your home to attend a meeting – video conferencing can bring everyone into your lounge room.

We are still of an age where children are computer savvy, leaving many adults lagging behind, the degree to which depends on the age of the adult. Presently, there exists a culture of some individuals knowing nothing else, some having some knowledge and others being irretrievably lost in the ever-evolving world of technology.

In the early 20th century, the invention of the television dominated many forms of leisure activities. It became a concern that too much time was spent in front of a screen, leaving less time spent on more productive and communicative based activities such as reading, playing games, getting involved in sports or hobbies, exploring, entertaining or being creative, singing, playing a musical instrument, drawing/painting, writing or some other form of innovative activity.

I am one of those adults who is middle range techno savvy and grew up in the time of only television and radio, before digital technology became a thing. As there wasn't much to keep us occupied indoors, we spent the majority of our leisure time outdoors. On our arrival home from school, we would quickly dump our bags, grab something to eat and scurry outside. It was a super let down if you happened to be home sick all day, laid up in bed, to hear all the squeals, laughter and merriment of the neighbourhood children signifying the end of the school day.

Books and comics weren't a substitute. The glee around the neighbourhood only dissipated as the children were ordered home at dinner time. Some parents would ring a bell, others would holler over back fences or send an errand child to summon their flock back home. After dinner, the family entertainment would continue in the lounge room, where we would huddle together on the couch and choose between two television channels. The choices were limited.

Although we were involved in "screen time" we were still very much involved in "child's play". We had our favourite programs and a lot of boring in-between stuff. This allowed us a wandering attention span, giving us the opportunity to talk, bicker, tease or tickle each other. We had a favourite television night. That was Sunday as there would be a movie playing. That was it. A time before video recorders and DVD players, let alone pay TV. Any other movies would require a visit to the cinema or drive-in to view.

A rotary dial phone lived in the hallway on a table with an attached seat. Tucked under the table was a phone directory which served as a contact list for telephone subscribers and a search engine for local businesses. As prestigious as an encyclopedia, the telephone book was a treasured household item, as it was the only go to place to find a contact and a platform for advertising. There was only one telephone in the household, so if it was in use, you would have to wait your turn. Public phone booths were commonplace for those who didn't own a phone. The only form of communication outside the immediate vicinity was by foot, car, telephone, telegram or mail delivered in the letterbox.

Before MacDonald's and KFC, the only take away was fish and chips and Chinese food. You would have to drive your own Uber and take your own containers to collect the Chinese which in those days before Tupperware were pots and pans from the kitchen cupboard.

And so, it was.

As time travelled forward it became a privilege for households to own more than one television, so the family began to segregate to varying rooms of the home to watch their preferred programs. Technology has advanced and it's not uncommon now for individual family members to own a multitude of screens that provide entertainment, connections to others and information on anything. Information that used to require a collection of encyclopedias or hours spent in a library to acquire. An internet search engine now provides updated information and data within an instant. Phones and watches have now become miniature computers with a multitude of functions.

There are many avenues now available that enable international correspondence. A few decades ago, we would have to choose an appropriate time to make an international phone call and wait days or even weeks for overseas mail. We socialised with those in our local communities, as we didn't have the means for our network to extend much further than that. Relatives and friends living some distance away, would be visited periodically when we had the means and time to do so. Nowadays, international communication is effortless. We can be in touch with anyone around the globe. There's no need to consider time zones or endure the lengthy wait it once took for reply correspondence to appear in the letterbox. Return correspondence from the other side of the world can be achieved in as little as 24 hours.

The fast-food industry has now saturated the planet, with thousands of restaurant chains cropping up all over the globe. Takeaway foods are now deliverable within minutes of placing an order. There's no need to leave home and tracking devices assess progress from restaurant to destination.

No longer dependent on members of the household for interaction and entertainment, technology has changed the character of human connections. There is now the opportunity for real people to communicate through online virtual characters (avatars) while gaming. These game buddies are role players in video games, interacting with other real people through their game playing avatars. Individuals connect online, sometimes for hours on end, playing with people with whom they are already socially acquainted or with strangers they only ever get to meet through their characters.

There are countless software applications accessible on computers, laptops, mobile phones and watches that enable people to connect to entertainment, shopping sites, banking, navigation, online forums and social media. Real life three-dimensional experiences are pushed aside in favour of the instant gratification attached to digital entertainment. It's fast, it's easy and it's interesting. There are endless opportunities as these apps keep populating. Unlike being involved in reading a book, watching a television program or listening to a radio, we can switch from one activity to the next within seconds on a computer screen without having to change devices.

Our brains aren't designed to effectively process two or more things at the same time. The brain needs to redirect focus from one thing to another, which requires concentration and time. With technology at our fingertips, we are more inclined to multitask, but this constant activity of switching from one task to another weakens our attention span, our clarity and our capacity for focus and deep thought. Overloading the brain with an avalanche of assorted information affects the normal pathways necessary for storing information to form memory.

In controlled measures, digital technology can be a great asset for learning and skill development in children. However, overexposure can stagnate physical activity and impact attention spans. A toddler's tantrum can be quickly fixed by handing over a technical screen. A parent's godsend, but this instant gratification deprives the child of learning how to self soothe, necessary for regulating emotions. Children can become so accustomed to digital entertainment and its associated addictive nature that they indulge in less indoor/outdoor play. They may forfeit missing out on activities which are important in exercising imagination and boosting creativity.

The mere pace of digital technology and the ability to multitask, can be quite taxing on the human brain, requiring thought processes to randomly switch circuits. Although a lot of information can be obtained in a short period of time and tasks can be accomplished quickly, this affects the mind's ability to engage in abstract thinking required for creative thought and problem solving.

When immersed in digital technology, we are removed from our senses, which connect us to ourselves, our surroundings and one another. This involvement suppresses the inner mind, preventing our thoughts and feelings a chance to communicate with us. Intuition is our higher consciousness, our connection to something greater than analytical thought. Our intuition brings forth answers. It props up the signposts guiding us through the maze of life. If we don't open up to it, we can become lost, frustrated and stressed, as we become more and more involved in our world of constant distractions.

Numerous distractions give us little, if any, time for reflection, in which we allow ourselves the time to listen to our inner mind speaking to us, amongst our randomly drifting thoughts. A disconnection to intuition can threaten peace of mind and we can become susceptible to anxiety and depression, joining the ever-growing queue for prescription medication.

Social media platforms have enabled universal connectivity. Not only is it a place where we can share our lives with others, we can seek community help, network, advertise and promote businesses, amongst other things.

Facebook is one of the most popular platforms and is a medium to share photos, updates and news with people who you have friended. There is a constant influx of stories and announcements on social media usually depicting the positive aspects of people's lives. News is shared, social encounters and holidays are publicised on screen.

Gone are the times of avoiding Aunt Betty with her newly developed photos of her overseas trip or luxury cruise. Now you just have to peruse Facebook and it's all there; cascades of pictures of your friends and acquaintances, partaking in life's pleasures. Whether you wanted to view them or not, there they are. Once you have taken a glance at who's posted on Facebook, you are compelled to keep scrolling. There's more: people involved in the glories of life, happy gatherings, happy family lives, on flights to exotic holiday destinations followed by an assortment of snapshots at these various locations, cocktails in the foreground, yachts in the background, enjoying life at its best.

These images are thrown into your world with no regard to your position in life at the time. Your life events may be on the other side of the spectrum at that same moment. If your life isn't going well, you may wish you could step right out of it and straight into their picture. You don't begrudge your friends their good fortune, however, it can sometimes make you feel their life is better than yours. An avalanche of stories depicting good times had by those other than yourself, can naturally conjure up envy and disappointment, particularly in times that are less than good for you. Their showy "happy" lives can accentuate any feelings of discontentment you may be experiencing and trick you into believing these people are living in luxury compared to the ordinary life you consider you have. It may seem these people don't have the worries and struggles you do.

Much of what is posted on Facebook is edited or glossed over. People usually post their "better side". We know this already, right? But before we realise, we have already reacted to the image portrayed. Photoshop allows you to conceal your less than perfect self, so the person framed in the destination of paradise matches it with a flawless complexion, great tan and perfect body. It's a shame the old polaroid photographic shots weren't able to perform the same magic. We used to rely on professional photographers to enhance our images, now we can do it with apps. The edited versions of ourselves and others posted on social media, are devoid of messy emotions and experiences. We all have failure, despair, struggles and anger that we don't put out for public consumption.

We have to remember behind the scenes. That the images captured on Facebook aren't a representation of reality and what we are viewing is just a portion of life in any one of these individuals. A portion that we too have experienced at one time or another in our lives. Maybe not the exact same experiences but, nevertheless, enjoyable occasions deriving an equal amount of personal satisfaction.

We all have unique experiences, so even if we were framed in the same picture, our own experience would differ to that person we have our arm around. Our enjoyment of the moment will depend greatly on our mood, past experiences and to what degree we are focused in the present.

Social media takes away the awkwardness of face-to-face communication, where we may stumble and splutter over our words, later regretting what we spilt out of our mouths. There is deliberation in what we communicate, allowing correction of such speech blunders. We can say anything we like without the embarrassment of reading what was just delivered through body language. There is an etiquette to behold in face-to-face communication. We have to meet with personal distances, interruptions, silences and the cues of body language. These signal what we can and cannot reveal and enable us to set the tone of our conversation. Face-to-face communication is a confronting complex process, much of which can be obliterated when communicating on social platforms. The security of communicating from behind a screen allows us to be a little more daring. In cyber land there are instant reactions and approvals to posts, whereas when contemplation and reflection take place, the desired response isn't always as forthcoming.

On the dating front, digital technology gives us the advantage of loosening the mask worn in the 3D world. First impressions can be glorified in the absence of initial face-to-face interactions. People can feel more at ease and take the time online to get to know one another before arranging a meeting. The means to seeking a potential partner is no longer reliant on friends, clubs or chance meetings. In fact, you can simultaneously date several people at one time. There are benefits and drawbacks to this method of dating. The stages of the relationship can propel forward at a quicker rate than in traditional dating and decisions on whether or not to pursue the relationship can occur prematurely with so many options available. The internet gives people an opportunity to connect with a lot of different types in a short space of time, which, in one sense, can be overwhelming and in another, providing such a wide selection allows for a better opportunity of finding a suitable partner. Once online dating shifts to face-to-face encounters, some foundations have already been laid, thus reducing the awkwardness that often accompanies those first dates.

Technology has brought us a long way forward. Communication, advertising and accessing information is so much easier than it once was. Entertainment is on tap. Boredom is a thing of the past. You could say that our ancestors lived a simpler life without the complexities of today's world. What are the advantages of then and now?

Way back, our ancestors lived off the land eating fresh produce they either farmed or hunted, built their own shelters and fetched fresh water from wells or streams. They were very much in tune with nature; they made their own medicine from plants and could accurately forecast the weather by surveying the activity of the birds and animals and by reading the sky. They would listen to sounds attuned to the land instinctively knowing when to hunt for food and when to run from prey. They sat, watched, listened and learned by utilising their intuitive antennas.

This lifestyle was non-sedentary. The villages were small. Travelling was limited. There was no pressure to conform or compete with others. Manual labour and outdoor living kept people exposed to good amounts of sunlight and fresh, unpolluted air. As the sun set, there was a drop in temperature and a campfire was lit. The only other illumination breaking through the blackness of the night, came from the moon and stars in the sky. Sleep came readily following an early rise and the physical activities of the day. There was no such thing as artificial light or lack of sunlight to upset normal circadian rhythms.

And now, we have the advantage of many job options. We can buy our fresh produce at convenience stores. Our shelters are built for us and we can choose where to live. We can travel wherever we want around the globe. Our communities are extensive.

There's no need now to rely on any in-built compass as we have meteorologists to predict our weather forecasts. The introduction of artificial light in the 19th century has allowed us to work and play well into the night. We no longer need to go to bed when night falls or wake around the same time the sun rises.

Our circadian rhythms are out of their natural sync and we tend to live on less sleep to fit more in, sometimes even finding it difficult to schedule in sleep. Alarm clocks are used to keep us on schedule, abruptly alerting our bodies to wake up, bypassing the natural, gentle sleep-wake cycle.

Technological advances have admittedly made our lives more comfortable and luxurious but not without a price. It has set up a more sedentary lifestyle and created more pressure to perform and compete with others. Unlike our ancestors, we are not reaping the benefits of physical exercise and exposure to sunlight, important in assisting our quality of sleep and immune function.

With the pressure and stress of a more complicated life, we may welcome shortcuts and choose fast foods over fresh produce. We favour driving over walking, mostly because it saves precious time, and tend to park as close to our destination as possible. We will even fritter away time driving around a car park to grab that "perfect spot". What is that all about?

Even though our lifestyles are different, we have not lost the skills of our ancestors. They just lay dormant. We are less in tune with our intuitive side and the natural rhythms of our body.

We are very focused on time as we feel we have little of it, which is true in our modern day fast-paced world. There's so much to do. Technology has allowed everything to be switched on 24/7. We rush around trying to fit everything in, as well as trying to maintain a healthy balance between work, family and social life. Our brains are often in multifunction mode, making it difficult to switch off and sit still. When we do have a free moment, we get busy in our heads; making sure to check in on the "to do" lists and pick up our worries from the day before. And if there is a temporary interval in between these thoughts, that space can be quickly filled by checking one of our "companion screens" for new emails or posts.

Our ancestors didn't have the distractions that we do. They had plenty of free time and lived alongside nature, which gave them room for intuitive downloads. We, on the other hand, have to make a conscious effort to free up time and create a suitable environment conducive to unveiling our sixth sense.

In order to bring back the skills of our ancestors, we need to free up time from our busy schedules and thought processes. To do this, we need to slow down, unplug from the pace of the world, prioritise what's important and what isn't and reset our body clocks to a state of balance and equilibrium. We need to feel comfortable in a state of boredom and give sleep back the time it deserves.

Simply immersing in nature or "forest bathing", calms the mind. You are probably already aware of how peaceful you feel when having a picnic in the park or a stroll along the beach. Here we are in our natural habitat, disconnected from the demands of the hustle and bustle of everyday living.

In a busy world interlaced with digital technology, there is less time for meaningful human connections. Partially because we are time poor and partially because we can bypass living in the three-dimensional world. To develop compassion and empathy we require real life interaction with other human beings. It requires being in touch with our feelings. The skills we require to identify our own feelings and to understand how others are feeling, comes from an inner knowledge we develop when we are involved in a functioning three-dimensional world. This inner knowledge often presents to us in a silent form. Body language cannot be revealed in a digital environment and so, there are missing pieces in the relationships we form online.

Periods of idleness, of doing nothing but just being, allow us to become attuned to our bodies, our thoughts, our senses and our impulses. Time spent in the virtual world desensitises us. We are no longer in touch with our sense of self and the connection we have with our environment. It is in being sentient that we tap into our inner thoughts and feelings and exercise our perceptions, thus creating a repertoire of memories. These memories thread into our life tapestry, enabling us to experience the past and the present in all of its intensity.

When tuned into technology, we are only fractionally present in life. It cuts into our ability to focus and really be present in life as it is happening. We have to be careful not to become tunnel visioned, oblivious to the real happenings occurring right around us.

As much as technology has made our lives easier, we need to maintain a healthy balance in our lives, otherwise we may risk stepping further afield from our innate abilities, the connections we form with our fellow humans and the elements and natural rhythms of our worldly surrounds.

EXPECTATIONS

If we could view our lives through a crystal ball, we would hope that futuristic ball would show a picture of health, happiness, success and a reasonably fair life with a selection of opportunities. We would hope to see longevity and good relationships within our life. We wouldn't want to miss out on parts of life that others get to enjoy. Life, we hope, will give us our fair share of pleasurable experiences and if it doesn't, it owes us!

Life is unpredictable and if we assume it will always turn out the way we want it to, we will undoubtedly be led to disappointment. Expectations shouldn't overshadow the joy of living. If things go differently to plan, you have simply scooped up an opportunity card. Accept it as a challenge. There is always something to be gained. You might even be surprised at how you handle a different-than-expected scenario.

If it were possible to see into our future, to know exactly what was ahead of us, would we be any happier or be in a better position in life? What if we saw something we didn't like? Would it take away our choices, our freedom? Isn't it the surprise factor, the unknown future that propels us forward? The same road travelled is boring compared to one not known. Right?

The good times in life are only made better because we have experienced the bad times. Life can get monotonous if expectations are always the same.

There are certain celebratory days; Christmas, Weddings, Graduations, Formals and the like, for which we carry high expectations. It would seem that fate would be playing a mean trick on us if anything was to ruin the day that was special. Still, the unpredictability of life occurs on any day, smashing the dreams of our presumed-to-be perfect day.

Every Christmas is the same but different. This is one day of the year universally celebrated. The meaning of Christmas comes from the birth of Christ but many non-believers still celebrate the day. Christmas is a time when people come together to bond, renew relationships, exchange gifts and indulge in festivities. It is anticipated to be a day of happiness, joy and fulfilment. It is a time to be grateful and to reflect on all the goodness in our lives.

Weeks, even months, before the most celebrated day of the year, preparations for the big festivity begin. It is difficult to ignore the atmosphere of gaiety and to not become involved in some way. Christmas becomes a popular topic of conversation in the workplace, amongst family and friends. There is a general buzz as people share their own exciting plans and a cheerfulness permeates the atmosphere. With all the built-up excitement, a great deal rides on what Christmas day is going to deliver.

The true spirit of Christmas is best experienced in the companionship of others. To be alone defeats the purpose of celebration as it is very much geared around sharing the special day with others. Every year, Christmas rocks up regardless of how it finds you. There is no pre-courtesy check in to see if your mood or situation is compliant with the gaieties about to besiege you. We all go through phases: good, bad and sometimes, just mediocre. Some years we will feel more festive than others. This could largely just depend on our mood of the day or it could be due to events in our lives that may either enhance or dampen our Christmas spirit. Like any day of the year, our mood will be reflective of our life situation at the time. Some days in our lives are difficult and some are easy, some days we are happier than other days and that's just the way it rolls.

Christmas does not discriminate and so we experience it according to where we are presently seated in life. There can be times in our lives when we don't feel like celebrating because of illness, grief, life events or isolation. Know that this is okay and there are other people that have similar struggles as well. Even those putting on a brave face. You may even be able to muster up enough courage to celebrate in a smaller way or bravely opt out altogether.

Just because you have experienced fabulous Christmases in the past, doesn't mean that these will repeat themselves each year. Some years are tough and you will be naturally inclined to just want to bypass the event. Christmas is a day that comes and goes and even when you have high expectations of how it should be, these expectations won't always be fulfilled.

It can be difficult to say "no" to invitations but being honest about how you are feeling will help others understand that you would prefer some quiet time. There is no point in pushing through the festivities just to please others, if it is in detriment to your wellbeing.

Commercialisation can take away from the true meaning of Christmas. The simplicity of gathering together and celebrating with the exchange of gifts and love can easily be blown out of proportion.

Looking back over the many Christmases I have had, there is a mix of good and average. As a child, every Christmas was pretty much the same. Staying at home on the day and enjoying family time. I came from a modest family, consisting of six members bordering on the poverty line. The most exhausted member of the family sat up late on Christmas Eve, in order to wait for a peaceful moment when all her children were bedded, including her husband, to wrap the Christmas presents.

My mother religiously hid these presents in a suitcase on top of her bedroom wardrobe. Little did she know that there were many years we'd scamper to the top of that wardrobe to discover the hidden treasures. My brother, the eldest and most mischievous, would be the last to bed and first to rise. Once he woke each sibling, the day would begin. Gathered in the lounge room, we would sit in quietness for a short while until excitement overrode a reasonable time to wake our parents.

Before long, the lounge room was awash with discarded wrapping. Mum would scurry around, retrieving and folding the bits of paper she could reuse next year. We had a short time to enjoy our gifts before donning on our very best outfits to attend church. On our return, we would pile our stack of presents into separate areas of the lounge room to be admired throughout the day, each of us secretly assessing the quality and quantity of gifts in each pile to be satisfied that all was fair and even.

We happily played with each other and our newly acquired possessions whilst enjoying the aroma wafting from the kitchen, as my mother busily prepared a special roast lunch. There were plenty of mishaps from year to year. Dad got too drunk on Christmas Eve, sometimes flaking it on the kitchen floor. Mum had many tizzy-fits as she felt the entire pressure of being the sole provider and peacemaker of the day. The house was wonky, as were the fixtures in it. The seal on the oven door was broken and many a time a chair was carefully propped against it to prevent it from slipping open. If that happened, which was often the case, the meal we expected at lunchtime wouldn't be ready until mid-afternoon. It didn't matter. When mum called, 'Ready,' we would rush to take our places at the kitchen table, last one in collecting the chair that attended to the oven and sit to devour the meal that had danced around our olfactory nerves for the last few hours.

Once mum sat at the table, often with the tea towel still flung over her shoulder, she could finally relax. All the preparation for Christmas was finally over for her. From decorating the Christmas tree, shopping, wrapping of presents, dragging dad from the kitchen floor, washing and ironing our Sunday best for church, to spending a good part of the day in the kitchen cooking and warding off anyone snitching food or wanting her attention before she could put her tools down.

Despite the misadventures, we always managed to enjoy the day because we were with our loved ones. As children, there was always the excitement of the gifts, but this was only a small part of it. There were times we still fought, although we tried to hold it together as it was sacrilegious to bicker on such a holy day and times, we felt a pang of envy when we discovered the neighbourhood kids out on the streets with their new sets of wheels. Bikes in our household were always reserved for birthday gifts and were second hand versions at that, usually spruced up with Dad's paintwork. What was captured more vividly in the memory bank on Christmas day was time spent with family.

The routine repeated itself year after year. We grew up to become adults, the family extended but the feel of the day was the same. We still kept our gatherings simple and found toys that suited all members. One particular year, Christmas day was a scorcher and a water fight commenced. This progressed over the years to become an annual water fight competition between our family members and that of our neighbours. Adults, children, toddlers, visitors. No one was exempt from a spray or saturation, if they ventured outside the sanctuary of the house or approached in the line of fire. It was a matter of how fast you could run. Buckets and hoses, water bombs and hand pistols soon gave way to super soaker guns and blasters, as the competition grew from year to year. The bigger, the better. And so it was, as we all gathered at 4 Skene Street.

As the family grew, it multiplied and dispersed, which now makes it too difficult for everyone to gather at the same location. Time is often divided so as many members of the family can get together for at least some part of the day's celebrations, but it usually costs hours spent on travel. Some members live too far away to join the extended group, some are unavailable due to work commitments and some settle for smaller gatherings with whoever can make it. At times our only connection is through phone greetings.

Commercialisation has the potential to spoil Christmas by increasing expectations of the day. Time and money are factors that may contribute to devaluing the simplicity of Christmas. Time can be spread too thin in an attempt to accommodate everyone, with a good chunk of Christmas day spent on travel so the event can be shared with extended family members. This may involve dividing the day into two or three sections. A meal at each location interspersed with road trips. And at the celebratory location, the host of the day's gathering often does most of the leg work behind the scenes. The one day of the year conducive to relaxation may just be an add-on to the pre-Christmas stress and weariness.

Stress and anxiety can accompany Christmas as expectations escalate and we work harder to earn more money or to free up time so we can step in line with everyone else. There seem to be more people to buy for every year. We have to spend substantial amounts on food as a feast is expected and also factor in travelling expenses. By heck, there's even more to be spent on decorations. The lit-up tree in the window is now amateur compared to the competing houses and streets. The contest gathers momentum to involve neighbourhoods and districts. God forbid the pressure you feel if you live in one of those illuminated areas!

We often carry an optimistic view of Christmas being the perfect day. We envisage others having that picture-perfect day portrayed in carols and movies. We see others carrying their numerous gift bags as they stroll happily along the beautifully decorated shopping malls, children sitting on Santa's knee, smiling for a family snapshot. Everyone blends into the lyrics of the overhead carols playing.

In our world, things may be different. At the same shopping centre, we may feel rushed, tired and agitated as we have nothing in hand, the carols playing grind on our nerves as we hurry through some last-minute shopping with an already maxed out credit card and little time left to purchase a few "just in case the cousin or neighbour gives me a gift" presents. Or we may have another scenario that is not particularly fitting with a joyous occasion.

The common mishaps in life still befall Christmas day

like any other. In the reality of everyday living, things never go perfectly. When you're supposed to feel happy and jolly and you put extra effort into feeling that way: early nights, biting your tongue to avoid arguments and putting worries and concerns on the back burner, you naturally have high expectations. These, however, may collide with reality causing disappointment and stress. If something goes wrong on what is supposed to be an unblemished day, its multitude is magnified.

Christmas rolls around at the end of each year, which signifies a time of reflection on the 12 months that have just passed: the events that have occurred, how we lived our lives and what our priorities were. We get ready to make some New Year resolutions and may have regrets in not having achieved the ones we made the previous year. A lot may have happened in the last year. Or nothing much at all. There will be times when we are proud of our achievements and other times when we feel frustrated and disappointed, as another year rolled by so quickly and time or commitment didn't permit us a chance to accomplish what we wanted.

Christmas is an example day in our lives when we have high expectations. Christmas comes and goes like any other day. Sometimes, it simply rains on our parade. There will be times our expectations will be met and other times not. Life is unknown and unlike being a character in a play, we cannot rehearse in order to perfect the scenes. The best we can do is alter the character we are playing.

PERFECTION

Wouldn't we all just love to have the perfect everything? Starting with our physical appearance, looks complimented by the flawless body, followed with a great home in a perfect location or, better still, several homes in various perfect locations around the world. These homes would have lush green gardens with a scattering of money trees. Let's add the career of our dreams, the perfect family and perfect friends and success in anything we put our golden hand to. Dream on.

    We are imperfect bodies in an imperfect world. Some people seem to have it all but that's far from the truth. Look at the rich and famous. Magazines, social media and newsfeeds glorify their looks and positions in life. It's easy to be tainted by the envy brush when we view the lives of these people. They live in luxury multi-million-dollar mansions, set in the most desired locations. They are usually very attractive and if they didn't start off this way, they have the money and artists to make them so. On the surface, celebrities appear to have it all. They may never have to worry about money and they live a comfortable lifestyle, but sacrifices have to be made to keep up their status. The main one is privacy. They are constantly followed by the paparazzi and have to share so much of their lives with the world.

There is always someone more attractive than us and someone less. Pretty faces tend to be symmetrical. It's not to say they are perfectly symmetrical but in better proportion to the average face. There are imperfections in even the most beautiful celebrities we know that may be well hidden, camouflaged with make up or corrected with surgery.

When it comes to beauty, most of us fall into the category of ordinary. The distinctively good looking and the less than ordinary make up the minority. We are exposed to beautiful people more than ever now, because technology has enabled imperfections to be erased. There are certain credentials that have to be met before embarking on a modelling career. Height, weight and attractiveness all need to meet certain standards. It can be similar in the acting industry, maybe not as stringent but attractiveness will certainly compliment skills. So, the people we view on screens and billboards are usually close to perfect. And we crave the same. Why wouldn't we when it's always in our face?

Our imperfections are a major marketing tool to lure us and sometimes scam us into purchasing various products and treatments. Cosmetic enhancements can make us look more attractive and younger than our true age. Let's face it, confidence can wane as the body ages and, as we are living longer, we need to feel comfortable in the skin we're in.

Some of us opt for aesthetic procedures to improve our body image, to look more appealing to the eye of the beholder and to improve our psychological wellbeing. If we look good, we feel good. And when we feel good about ourselves, more opportunities open up to us. There is such a wide selection of cosmetic treatments available, both surgical and non-surgical, to boost our confidence if that's our choice. However, for those of us not so favourably swiped with the genetic wand, there are other ways to improve our image.

We all have a body image. There are parts of ourselves that we like and other parts we would like to improve on. We tend to place more focus on our imperfections. And remember, everyone has them, even the most beautiful models whose photos are airbrushed by the way, although it is easy to forget this fact when we are struck by eye boggling beauty. We should try picking out our best features and focus on those. It's not all about physical appearance. We view ourselves in the mirror every day, so we get used to what we see. Other people's perceptions of us are usually favourably different to our own. We are judged on the whole of our persona. So, take into account the way you groom yourself, carry yourself, your personality and your strengths. Stand tall; don't slouch. Dress to accentuate your qualities. Smile a lot. Rock that body language. That's it. Confidence will overshadow imperfections. Hands down.

Once we get to know a person, their physical characteristics diminish as their inner substance is revealed. Let's face it, who hasn't met a drop dead gorgeous human specimen whose image has come crashing down once their personality has been revealed? Conversely, what of the plain Jane whose character overshadows any flaws in her appearance? Who would you prefer to be around? Besides, depending on the glasses we don for the day, we may idolise someone who, in another's eyes, is no more than ordinary.

Self-esteem is an integral part of our self-image. If we look good, we naturally boost our self-confidence and, if our confidence is up there, we have a better footing in life. It is important to get it right in those impressionable years when self-awareness and ego are emerging. If there are areas that need improvement such as braces to correct a smile or the treatment of acne, then it is best to take measures to correct self-image, before that image gains momentum in causing detriment to its wearer's persona.

It is human nature to measure up against others, so if we are constantly bombarded by perfect images, we are more likely to scan ourselves to seek out our imperfections. The more beauty around us, the more meticulous we will be in our own assessments. Beauty is powerful. Cosmetics, surgery and photography can obliterate imperfections. Eventually, youth and beauty give way and all of us, including those committed to their outward appearance who undertake extreme measures to always appear young and beautiful, will inevitably have to succumb to age.

Being obsessed with our packaging only ignites an endless preoccupation with appearance. Appearance is only transient. The true essence of our being: our soul, our spirit, our consciousness or whatever you like to call it, is what we carry through our existence, unhampered by ageing or physical imperfections. Live as the person from within, as the best external appearance won't substitute for an empty shell.

Social media sites have given us a platform to airbrush our persona. We can exaggerate our image to near perfection, covering up our weaknesses and failures. If we can live in a cyber-world portraying this fake image, how then do we reveal our true selves in the real world? Are we in danger of substituting real life relationships, by relying on the internet to constitute a social medium in which we can free ourselves of imperfections? As we have control over what we post, selecting and editing, we can portray a glorified online self, neatly tucking away our personal baggage. Will this then eventually lead to disconnection from what is real?

People who are perfectionists set their standards high, with little tolerance for human error. We all know that travelling toward our goals can be a bumpy ride and sometimes a longer journey than anticipated. As children, we are introduced to fairy tales with stories tending to end in the happily ever after, only to grow up to discover that life doesn't exactly roll out that way. If only we could have bottled Prince Charming and Fairy Godmother. Oh, and a superhero wouldn't have gone astray!

There is nothing wrong with trying to achieve high standards or to work to the best of our ability, as long as we are adaptive to what is good enough. Unforeseen events can cause a diversion in timelines and, if we allow for this, we can reset our goals without becoming flustered and feeling like a failure. Of course, if we are working toward a deadline, such as sitting an exam, then we can factor in more time to allow for these possible setbacks. Disappointment can so easily be avoided if we have realistic expectations and don't push ourselves beyond these.

There is a risk of becoming burnt out in the quest of working too hard or juggling too many things in an attempt to be good at everything. Set measurable goals. Allow yourself some slack. Sometimes you don't feel well enough or in the mood to keep ploughing ahead. Time out can reset and make you more productive when you resume your project or task. Sometimes you just won't get it all done in a day. Even if you have the time. Sometimes you simply bite off more than you can chew.

We're not superhuman beings that can multitask and get everything done efficiently in a set time, no matter how hard we try. Prioritising and accounting for miscalculated and interrupted time frames is a more realistic goal and one which could potentially avoid a headache that may otherwise greet the end of the day. Things happen. Don't pack your day full of tasks. Leave some room for the unavoidable interruptions in life.

Happiness is a state in which we would prefer to reside. Right? To be wrapped in a bubble of positive emotions: joy, gratitude, love, excitement and contentment as they make us feel good. Way more desirable than having to deal with any negative emotions: sadness, anger, loneliness, jealousy and fear, that bring us down. As it is in our makeup to experience a mixed bag of both positive and negative emotions, it is best to be amenable to all of them.

It is socially acceptable to express the positive emotions and keep a lid on the negative. How can this be fair when we weren't designed to be perfect beings? Isn't it good and right to express all emotions, in order to maintain a healthy psychological wellbeing? Untruths readily slip off our tongues when people greet us with, 'How are you?' The 'Good thanks,' or 'Well thanks,' responses aren't always appropriate but we dish them out anyway. These are acceptable responses that ease us through the greeting process, shoving any unsavoury emotions back down under the surface where they sit disguised, lest we scream them out.

The truth of how we are really feeling stays under wraps, left to fester until such a time that we feel in a safe place to spend time out, talk it over, shed a few tears or let holler. We have all experienced those crazy-arse horn honkers, even been culprits ourselves (my hand is up...g u i l t y!) throwing tantrums in their cars. It eventually all becomes too much when, whoa, a full bag of bad day emotions suddenly explodes. Negative emotions can cause an eventual spill-over, causing a bigger disruption than they would have, had they not been contained in the first place.

Perhaps, if we weren't conditioned to restrain the unpleasant emotions, they wouldn't be offensive and make others feel uncomfortable. If all emotions were accepted equally, they could be expressed accordingly and we could go about our lives free of the pent-up anger and frustration some of these suppressed emotions cause. Give all emotions the rights they deserve.

Part of living the fantasy of a fairy tale, a perfect life, is the desire to have it all. With this, comes the desire to make more money to be able to afford those items believed will improve our image and social status. We strive for more possessions, more exotic vacations, a career promotion and, to add a feather to the cap, even aspire to rub shoulders with those who are already icons through success and wealth. No matter how hard you endeavour to be equal to or better than, someone will always set the bar higher than you can achieve. There's no gain in working longer hours and "busting your balls" to afford the best of the best and keep up appearances, just to fall off the perch through pure exhaustion. What would be the point of that?

Perfectionism doesn't account for failure, which is an unavoidable part of our human existence. Failure is an integral stepping stone toward success. It is all a part of the learning process. A baby doesn't suddenly stand up and master the art of walking straight away. There will be numerous stumbles and falls. Throughout life we often fail before we succeed and these failures not only teach us valuable lessons, they are the catalysts for developing virtues such as kindness, empathy and compassion. Fearing failure can close the doors on success. People often believe failure is a weakness that gets in the way of success and is thus something that should be avoided. This is limited thinking. The most successful people owe their achievements to the many failures that preceded their accomplishments. The more times you pick yourself up from falling, brush yourself off and move forward, the more you take with you toward achieving your future goals. Failure gives us a greater appreciation of arriving at success; it makes us more confident, smarter and stronger.

If everyone was perfect, there would be no variety, no quirky. Instead, there would much sameness. And if that was the case, wouldn't our standards of acquiring perfection increase? Wouldn't we be aching to be a little different, a little unique? How else would we stand out from the crowd, identify with our individuality? If we complied with the image portrayed as the ideal human, there would be more pressure to change who we really are. What if you were the perfect human specimen living amongst a population of trolls, as in the movie, Shrek? Then I guess you would feel like a misfit and want to change to better blend in with the majority. I'd say it is better to stick with a bag of liquorice all sorts.

COMPARISONS

Who's taller? Who has the fuller glass of lemonade? Who can run faster? These are the quests of children. We grow into adults and make comparisons regarding who is making the most money, who has the better house, spouse, kids, career etc.

Comparing ourselves to others is a natural process. It is how we learn. It is how we define our status in life. It is important that we blend in and conform to society. There is societal pressure to behave in an acceptable manner and so we need to match our behaviours and attitudes to those around us. We have certain rules and etiquette to follow. We need to demonstrate punctuality, dress in appropriate attire, display table manners and stick to time schedules. If we don't abide by these rules, we are deemed rude and disorderly. And so, we behave in a social manner that is expected of us in order to fit in, to feel included and to become a part of the bigger picture that transforms us from a lone wolf to part of the pack.

Sometimes conforming to society involves peer group pressure. We form behaviours and adapt our attitudes and habits that are suitable to the pack we belong to. We want to feel that we are accepted within the group, because ultimately, we are social beings and it is important to interact and establish relationships in life. The need to feel included in a group starts at an early age and continues throughout life. The pressure to conform peaks during a time when we are most impressionable; the teen and early adult years when we are still forming our identities. This is a time we want to experiment with some of the "cool" or "socially acceptable" activities that others do, without much consideration given to the consequences or appropriateness of such behaviour. Opinions and choices are sometimes influenced by how we determine others will judge us and so we conform to what we believe to be socially accepted. As we mature and acquire a repertoire of life experiences, our self-image strengthens and we don't feel the need to conform so much. However, it is important for us to observe and follow other people's behaviours to determine our place in the world and to teach us valuable lessons on what works well for us and what doesn't.

We compare ourselves to those we feel superior to and those we feel inferior to. One feeds the ego and the other feeds our insecurities. The rating we give ourselves will either highlight our qualities or underestimate them. Accepting that there is and will always be someone better off and someone worse off than ourselves, will help keep us aligned with the strengths and qualities we possess. Strengths and qualities that we all have, irrespective of our personal rating.

When life seems unfair for us, it is easy to compare our lives to others and assume theirs is better. We know our lives inside out. We cannot know others' lives so intimately. To those with whom we are close, we do get a bit more of an inside glimpse, but unless we live in another's shoes, we can't presume they got dealt a better pack of life cards. Comparing our lives with others is futile. What appears to be a better life for others is just our own perception. When we are envious of someone else's possessions or position, we are most likely looking through a distorted lens. We often choose a higher-than-average benchmark. We pull out our pens, paper, calculators and rulers to meticulously tally up what that person has that we don't. Whatever it is: success, a freer lifestyle, more assets or numerous other possibilities, it will only lead us down the path of dissatisfaction. One of thinking we aren't good enough or could do better. This mentality blinds us to the attributes we already possess, those that, unbeknown to us, others secretly envy.

In comparing yourself to others and what other people have that you don't, is just a waste of time. Valuable thinking time wasted on someone else's life instead of your own. Wouldn't it be better to focus that energy on investing in your own life path; the one you have a personal vested interest in? You are where you are right now in life. You can revisit your past but you can't change it. You can instead, be grateful for what you have and be excited on how you want to move forward in creating your future. Embrace your past as it has been a catalyst in the making of the person you are now. Without the mistakes, hurts and losses you wouldn't have developed the strength and adversity that you have today. So be proud.

When you find you're comparing yourself to others, do it in a productive way, taking away something positive that you can apply to your own life. Other people may give you the incentive to try harder, take up a new project or polish the qualities you already possess, discover new ones or change your direction in life. All of which will empower you. Look out for these gifts. Believe in yourself. Practise collecting attributes that you find attractive in other people and apply them to become a better version of yourself.

What appears to be a more perfect world: glamour, glitz, beautiful people partaking in perfect lives is only a façade. One that is constantly in our faces. If not in the real world, there in the cyber world. Reality is camouflaged by the ability to cover up the ugly parts. Once upon a time a model showcased on a billboard may have created a touch of envy, but it was known to be a propped image enhanced by all the editing; a skill reserved for professional photography. Now, social media showcases the best of everyday people looking great and living the dream life and we are left to wonder why we don't have the looks and fairy tale life of others. Even though our brains may be aware that what we are actually viewing is just the favourable parts of others' lives and photoshop software has enhanced the picture, we have already subconsciously jumped into making comparisons, well before our reasoning mind has a chance to dispute that line of thinking.

Lives are messy for everyone. We all have bad hair days and much worse than that. It's just that this messiness occurs at different intervals in life for everybody. We don't exist on parallel planes, so our ups and downs don't occur simultaneously to others. Whilst one person is experiencing a good moment there is guaranteed to be another experiencing a bad moment and vice versa. Life is full of hurdles; we all have to jump them.

Celebrate your uniqueness. Consider this: In the vastness of the universe, we are one very small speck. Like sand on the seashore, we are a part of what makes up the whole. Each grain is a different size, shape and colour and yet it blends altogether to create the floor of the sea and shore. In the scheme of things, we are a very small part of the tremendous greatness of the universe. We live on one of the planets called Earth, which narrows us down in the immensity of the galaxy. On this earth, we live in one of the 195 countries and within that individual country we live in one of the divisions, known as a province, region or state. We have the ability to travel around the globe but not around the galaxy. However, a good part of our lives is spent within our segregated communities, moving back and forth for work, family and social commitments and recreational activities. Those few people that live in existing tribal communities or in isolation, have an even more limited community and travel circumference.

There is a sense of detachment when peering out of the window of an airplane after take-off. As it ascends into the sky, the landscape below becomes smaller and smaller. People on the ground look like a scattering of ants. Cars, streets, houses, buildings, paddocks and lakes all begin to appear uniform, all combined as one and, as the plane continues to climb, everything disappears behind a blanket of cloud. If we could look down on earth from a spacecraft, this feeling of detachment would be magnified and we would identify with our one entity as being rather inconspicuous. Just like a grain of sand on the seashore, miniscule, yet very much an integral part of all creation. With this perspective, we are able to step out of ourselves and appreciate the view that we are just a small portion of this wondrous universe.

When we are ground bound, it is easy to have a limited vision of just our immediate surrounds and an awareness of our being as a separate entity and not a part of a unity of oneness. In other words, it is easy to fathom living within the confines of our narrow view. Like organisms confined to a petri dish, we can't see beyond our boundaries. There is a greater intelligence than ours working in harmony to maintain our existence. We have no conscious control over how our heart beats and to what rhythm, nor can we direct which cells to eliminate and which to renew. Our bodies just know. Millions of our cells die and are replaced every minute throughout our lives. Who directs that? The earth provides gravity, sunshine, water and food to sustain us, all of which without we wouldn't be able to survive. Call it what you will: a greater power, the universe or God. There is a divine intelligence synchronising everything. We are in control of some things, we do have free will, but there is a bigger player in our lives. Once this is realised, we are more able to disengage from our self-importance and concentrate on living a life without being competitive or envious of one another.

Our lives are segments of moments all connected together to form the totality of our existence. As humans, we are always interconnected with mankind, one in all, sharing the same life energy. Our forms are different at varying times through age and experience but we are all on the same life game board. Individuality should be accepted as well as embraced. Each of us has a part to play which contributes to the growth, harmony and wellbeing of the whole: in work, relationships, family and society. We all have something to teach one another, allowing the wheels of the universe to keep turning. Instead of judging appearances and behaviours in others and comparing them to your own, use them as tools to learn from or just appreciate the varieties that make life the intricate tapestry it is.

As much as the universe is complex as it is vast, we are in flow with it. We are all, at this very point in time, on our own life path. Let go of comparisons. We all have similarities and differences to others on this same planet. That will never change.

PART THREE

● ● ● ●

Importance of Time

LIVING IN THE PRESENT

In this game of life, we are given a certain amount of time. Our aim is to utilise this time in the best way possible and to keep moving forward in the hope that we have plenty of forward moves before our time runs out. Sometimes we lose a few turns. Missed opportunities. Sometimes we get stuck in the same position and don't move at all. Procrastination. At other times, we focus on time that has passed and time ahead of us, which interferes with the time we are in at present. Stagnant. Although we cannot physically backtrack, we can mentally retrace our previous moves to make smarter decisions on the way forward. The exact amount of time we have in life is not disclosed to us. We have to make the most of the time we have at present.

The way in which we spend our time will have a huge influence on our life experiences. We have all been issued time keys. These keys give us a choice on what life episodes to open and how much time we spend in each of these episodes. The keys will only work in the present. We can't go back and unlock time in the past or prematurely use these keys for future purposes. We can, however, allocate and set aside keys to use in the future. All we should carry on our person are the keys we can use for now, the present. With so many keys it is sometimes difficult to distinguish the ones for present use. Our brains tease us with so much backward and forward thinking that we sometimes leave the keys in our pockets and miss the events of now. Or we may open episodes but don't fully engage in them.

Prioritising what is important can help keep us living as intended: in the moment. So much time can needlessly be wasted when we are too preoccupied to be able to engage in the present. It could be because we are caught up in our heads, in meeting deadlines or simply rummaging in a bag to find a camera or phone, to take a picture or record the event in which we are partaking. All of these disruptions can interfere with the full enjoyment of the moment. It is fabulous to have a recording to reminisce over when the present becomes the past, but if we are viewing the whole event through a camera lens then we are missing the bigger picture. Whatever it is we are experiencing in life, we will reap the benefits by being fully immersed. The authenticity and grandeur of an event can be diminished if we are only partially engaged.

Many of us, let me just take a stab in the dark and say, all of us, have at one point or another missed or minimised our experiences, because of our preoccupation with thoughts that swing from past to future, only intermittently pausing to focus on the present. Of course, we do have to step out of the moment from time to time to reflect on the lessons of past experiences and the future consequences of our present actions, so we don't behave inappropriately or recklessly. Once these assessments have been made, we can release all mind chatter and distractions and connect on a conscious level where our senses meet the physical world of now.

In search of something else, something better, the moment in the present may be disregarded in the hope of a better moment in the future. All we have is the moment. We can envisage future moments but they are only how our mind imagines them to be. They aren't tangible right now. The moment slips away and it is soon past as further segments of moments come into being. Our life is one perpetual cycle of moments. As we go for a stroll, how can we be totally absorbent of the warmth of the sun on our clothes and the gentle breeze wisping through our hair or the greenness of the trees and the cloudless blue sky, if our thoughts are tied up with yesterday and tomorrow?

Some may think that being engrossed in the moment might eliminate success and growth in life, that instead of being passive in the now, time should be spent planning ahead. When you think about it, when you infuse yourself in the present, you become more aware, more connected, which enables a more concentrated focus on everything you do in life. Isn't that the definition of success? Not dilly dallying in your subconscious mind full of what was and the what ifs, that you have no control over. All you need to take from the past is what you have learned and the memories that have brought you to where you are today. You can be in control of how you are thinking, which will influence how you feel. Savour the moment. Really live in it.

Seldom are any of us fully immersed in the present. This we can tell by our minds continually mulling over time. But what is time? Isn't it just a man-made measure to track our lives and put them into some sort of perspective? Time is really just an illusion. Past and future don't exist right now. We can't presently live in them! Right now, all we have is this moment in time. This moment houses our existence. Concerning ourselves with the concept of time that is to come or time which has preluded this moment, prevents us from extracting all that is available to us in the present. And if we can't engage all our senses in what we are experiencing right now, then we aren't able to live life to the fullest. Later, when one moment rolls into another, we may harbour regrets, feeding our mind travel and once again preventing us from being fully present in the current tense. A perpetual cycle of distraction can predominate our daily living.

To accept that there is a natural impermanence in all things in life is to allow a greater appreciation of what is now. It is the nature of things to change. Physical objects break or perish. Living things inevitably cease to exist. Nothing stays the same. As the clock ticks, the moment changes. A leaf falls from a tree, objects collect a new fleck of dust and since you read the last paragraph, your body has replaced several million cells. The universe gives to us and takes from us and so, it is futile to think we can truly possess anything. It is better to appreciate what we have in the world of now, as with the continuum of time it will at some point fail to exist.

People who are fully present in the moment are easy to be around. They are totally engaged in life, living exclusively for today. They bathe themselves in all they can extract from their surrounds and, as they are in flow with life as it happens, they are generally happier as thoughts don't interrupt their presence. Able to devote their full attention, they listen and interact well with others, they are emotionally available, which makes forming relationships with them so easy. Being able to anchor awareness in the here and now deepens relationships, contributing toward a more satisfying life.

Many of us take the present moment for granted, expecting that many of the same moments in life will be repeated. The consistency of everyday life may trick us into ignoring what we have in hand. Ask any parent who has raised a child, how many regrets they have as they inadvertently let many precious moments slip by during the transient passage of childhood. Ordinary daily events can be missed when we redirect our focus elsewhere. Think about what you've missed and what isn't as vivid in your memory because you lacked concentration on a time that is now past. Never to be regained.

Connecting with life as it presents to us is the healthiest way of living. With all the extra sensory stimuli present in today's busy world, it is difficult not to be distracted. The constant stimulation of our five senses triggers our thought processes, infiltrating our brains with a multitude of things to think about. Each of these cascading thoughts has an emotional attachment which affects our mood and the degree of presence we feel in the moment. Mindfulness is a state in which you are totally focused on what you are sensing and feeling in the moment, being aware of your thoughts and feelings without the distraction that they cause. Practising mindfulness helps keep us in the present. It has a calming effect, silencing thoughts of anxiety and regret often associated with mind travel. These negative thoughts have the tendency to alter our biochemistry, displacing our equilibrium, which can ultimately lead to associated health consequences. Mindfulness connects us to the moment. It has a therapeutic benefit in improving our psychological wellbeing.

To be in constant pursuit of goals and dreams for the future, in the hope that they will lead to the satisfaction we crave, is futile. Once there, the satisfaction fades and so we go in search of something else to chase, expecting that next thing to lead us to lasting satisfaction. Disappointed once again, we discover that this type of fulfilment is short lived. Why is this a surprise to us? Hadn't we already determined this, over and over? Before we know it, life is quietly creeping past and we have been so preoccupied in planning the future that we miss simply living in the moment.

The best way to work toward your future goals is to focus on what steps you need to take right now. Right now, is where you'll ever be. It is where you once were in the past and where you will again be in the future. Open yourself up to being satisfied in life now. Infuse yourself with all that you can take from the moment to bring about the future you desire. When you are completely receptive to your present surrounds, you will be able to engage all your senses, enriching your life and creating a happiness that is based on the gratitude of what you have right here in the now. Reap the benefits of now to take you into your tomorrow.

Have you ever been so involved in something that you realise you are oblivious to time or others around you? Being in flow is defined as: a mental state in which a person performing some activity is fully immersed in a feeling of energised focus, full involvement and the enjoyment of the process of the activity. It is a state in which a person is completely involved and focused on what they are doing, beyond the point of distraction. Where there seems to be a fluidity between mind and body. Many of us liken it to being "in the zone". When in flow, we are living in the moment utterly absorbed in the present activity. Time seems to slip away without us even noticing it and, for once, our head is clear of any intrusive thoughts. In this state of mind and body connection, we are able to filter out all distractions as thoughts synchronise together to perform the task at hand. There is a general feeling of serenity, wellbeing and fulfilment reported when in flow. This has to do with the complete absorption in a challenging task requiring our undivided attention. When self-awareness fades away, so too do the usual culprits of distraction: emotions, hunger, pain and lethargy, unable to disrupt our internal equilibrium. When a wandering mind is shut down there is a heightened sense of awareness activating natural pleasure producing and performance enhancing chemicals. Being in flow is an ultimate state of living in the present moment. Although flow is mostly a positive condition to reside in, there are manufactured experiences that feel like flow. Being involved in video gaming and gambling can shut out the world, creating the same loss of self-consciousness that the authentic version of flow produces. It's best to choose activities that create long term satisfaction, challenging enough to produce self-improvement and within a reasonable time frame so as not to sabotage real time required for relationships and commitments.

It is important to file our memories so we can reflect on our past lives and intertwine them with what is our present. Memory is the ability to be able to retrieve information that has been encoded and stored in the brain. To remember something requires recalling information from the past. A mental impression is retained of facts, events and experiences and filed to be retrieved when required. Retention of information is required to be able to develop language and personal relationships. It is essential for self-identity.

We are constantly laying down memories from our experiences. Whether they are remembered vividly or not, will depend on: the foundations of the memory, our emotional attachment and whether that memory is recalled from a near or distant past. There are some events we will remember more than others, depending on what attention we gave the newfound experience, what was happening around the time of the memory formed and how the experience influenced our emotional state, if at all.

What if we had no memories and each day we lived was a total new experience? We wouldn't have a sense of self or of how we came to be. Our own personality traits wouldn't be known to us. Would we even have a personality? After all, to develop distinctive traits would require recollection of data on a frequent basis and being able to retrieve information from past experiences. Our senses would be overwhelmed as we wouldn't recognise any of the smells, sounds, taste and sensations that we have become accustomed to. We'd meet everyone for the first time again and again and speak our minds with no conscious effort of filtering words or withholding information to suit the moment.

Life would always be new, always surprising. We wouldn't have a past as we wouldn't remember it. And if we couldn't remember a past, we wouldn't have any perception of a future, as thoughts about a future are greatly determined by past occurrences. The mind wouldn't have any cluttered shelves of stored information. It would be like an empty room, temporarily furnished with the day's events and quickly vacated again to become unoccupied. Data lost as soon as it was gained.

The present moment would be our total focus as there would be no past to reminisce or have regrets over and no future worries to contend with, as these usually stem from known experiences. The mind would remain untainted. No distracting mind chatter disturbing our presence in the moment at hand. Everything would be experienced in full appreciation. We would be totally in sync with the three-dimensional world.

If we had no memory, we would more likely be in a positive

state of mind, in wonderment of all that is in the moment. In the present is where we would always reside. We'd have no hang ups. No regrets. No fear. If anyone hurt us it wouldn't matter as we wouldn't remember the insult. Anger and resentment wouldn't exist.

Our memories are important to us, so it is important to create some good ones and carefully file them. We will recall memories more readily when we have an emotional attachment, so if you want to hold onto something special, utilising all of your senses can help you with this. Capture as much as you can in the moment; to help you later locate files you have subconsciously stored in your memory bank. This involves being as present as you can be in the moment. A journal, diary and pictures can all assist in retrieving memory files, keeping them vivid. Memories serve us well. They connect us to the people we know and the events that have shaped our lives.

We can be too preoccupied with time, focusing on timeframes and how long we have to complete a task, that we either forget, are unaware, or have no consciousness of "now". To just be in the present tense. Consider your "dream world" where there are no time constraints. You are perfectly involved in the present happenings as your dream plays out. Think of how it is when you reflect back on a dream and try and practise being focused like that in your "awake time", purely and utterly present.

Reactions to life are determined by our thinking. If you woke up from a dream disgruntled because your feelings were carried over from sleep time, you would be quick to dismiss them as they serve you no purpose in your awake world. Get back to the present. Why not dismiss all thoughts that don't serve you in the present just as quickly as you would leave a dream behind in your sleep world?

Shake off thoughts of past and future living. Now is the only time you have at present. There is no past to exist in, as it's just that, past or what was. There is no future to exist in, as it hasn't yet manifested. Life is right now. Jump in!

A WASTE OF TIME

We are always busy in our daily lives and then when we have free time, we feel we should busy it up with something lest we get bored or fritter away "precious time". Apart from catching up with what we have on our to-do-list, a hobby, interest, friends and family and social events, there are plenty of other activities to prevent boredom setting in. That spare minute can easily be consumed in screen time, emails to read and write, social media to peruse, news to catch up on, movies to watch and games to play. A dull moment no longer exists, let alone a moment of silence. A moment of nothing.

Leisure time isn't necessarily restful as it once used to be. There are many activities to fill in voids. There was a time before computer screens, before android phones and before android phones gave birth to android watches, a time even before television and radio, a period of time in which the brain was allowed to sit in pause mode. Technology has changed that. It has enabled us to switch from one set of stimuli to another in a matter of milliseconds, which requires the brain to perform some quick adjustments. When we multitask or quickly switch from one task to another, the brain is busy at work, shooting electrical currents from one neuro circuit board to another and, at the same time, frantically adjusting impulses to the numerous incoming signals. Filling in every square inch of time by keeping the mind occupied with "screen stuff" hot wires the brain.

Imagine tiny telephone switchboard operators inside your head, plugging and unplugging cables all over the place, working relentlessly and getting cranky because there's no time to take a break. With a multitude of incoming data, signals scramble everywhere. Not only do these signals have to be decoded to something recognisable by the brain, they stimulate a certain mood/feeling depending on the chemical reactions they activate. Just as the brain dissects one message, another comes through. The feel-good calming effect driven by the neurotransmitter, dopamine, may suddenly be knocked out by its rival neurotransmitter, norepinephrine, as it takes precedence, increasing alertness and heart rate. So, a feeling of relaxation may quickly convert to one of anxiety in a matter of seconds depending on how frazzled the cable workers get.

Our moods change according to the biochemistry of the brain. One moment you may be reading an interesting article on Google when pop up ads, cookies or notifications interrupt your flow. Immediately, your biochemistry takes a shift and you may find yourself annoyed, as not only have you been rudely interrupted, you have succumbed to multitasking. Let's just take a look at that ad or notification for a second, then go back to the article. Back at the article, there are links throughout, so you click on those so as not to miss anything. Pages further into all of the links, you attempt to get back to the article. Where the hell were you? Alas, you lost it. In frustration, you search through Google again, diverting your eyes for a quick moment to glance at the time and are surprised to notice just how much of it has passed.

Out of curiosity, even a sense of urgency, we feel compelled to draw away from what we are presently engaged in to open up links and notifications. It is a part of how technology plays us. There is some invisible intelligence pulling our strings with an uncanny knowledge of what keeps us engaged. The cable operators are the puppets, rearranging the connections to download software from device to brain. The brain soon overloads with an influx of information overriding its natural abilities, consequently affecting mood, memory and attention span.

The brain has no way of telling what is real and what isn't. You may have noticed a physical reaction to whatever the mind perceives as being real. This is known as the mind-body connection. Have you ever noticed how tense you become when you watch a thriller or horror movie or how a drama may bring out your emotional side? Well, interruptions to an activity your mind is engaged in, may have similar effects. Not only does the interruption pull you aside from what you were involved in, it may alter your emotional state.

The brain needs a time of stillness, a time of relief from perpetually tackling one task and swiftly switching to another. The motherboard requires time out so the brain can sit in neutral for a while, as it is only then it has the space to sort and stack information it has previously erratically shelved. The busier the brain is, the less time it has to clean up files and so, these files clutter up, occupying creative space. In order to clean up dumped information, file it properly and make some sense of it, the brain needs a break. Time out.

Brain respite occurs when we are in a state of complete relaxation. How many great ideas or resolutions come to you as you lay in your bed at night awaiting sleep? It may happen in the middle of the night or in the morning after sleep when the brain has completed yet another shift of sorting files, freeing up space to occupy new data. Permitting time to let our thoughts just wander allows for reflection, imagination and creativity.

Meditation allows respite for the brain. Indulging in a place in nature, whether it be just sitting quietly on the beach staring out into the ocean or strolling through a park, can have a tremendous effect on our state of mind. Normal concerns dissipate as we become attuned with nature. It's where we feel peace, solace, an innate connection, as once, that was all our surrounds ever was, before technology took hold of our environment and interrupted our state of being.

Filling in voids of time may stir up a whole lot of neurotransmitters that aren't conducive to a relaxed state of being. In our "leisure time" we tend to choose activities that give us a sense of productivity. As there is too little time to get everything done, we use some of our down time to complete tasks. Having "nothing to do" feels uneasy when there are so many things to fill time with. We can so easily become accustomed to ongoing mental stimulation, that it seems a sin to not occupy the mind with something.

In order to free up the mind, we need to step away from tech and other activities long enough to feel bored. The brain needs to dismiss the cable workers, pull up a recliner and chill out. A time to daydream and reflect and be at peace. This down time unlocks our thoughts and emotions, which are, much of the time, suppressed by the flurry of activity we are continuously engaged in. When we allow our mind the time to daydream, we are more in tune with our senses and our thoughts and emotions are left to wander freely, unlocking our productive and creative abilities. The brain gets back to its own unique talents of problem solving, making plans and designing ideas, all of which add purpose and meaning to life. So, what may seem like a waste of time is, in fact, time well spent.

SPONTANEOUS QUIET TIME

As life is filled with endless options to occupy the mind, it is difficult to acquire quiet time in which to tune into our inner being and the magnificence of our innate mental processes. To establish a connection with our thoughts, feelings and imagination, we require some unoccupied mind space.

Have you ever arrived earlier than anticipated for an appointment and felt a sudden sense of panic when you realise you have left your playmate (phone) behind and, apart from a few outdated magazines (boring), you have nothing to fill the void? As a reformed smoker, I remember that exact same sense of panic if I had left for the day without my pack of ciggies. Why is that? Each of these vices trigger our reward centres, flooding our brain with dopamine, pleasantly pacifying the mind.

Periods of boredom are more infrequent than they once were. In one respect, that's good as we needn't sit in a state of boredom for too long. On the other hand, it's not so good, as we require periods of nothingness to unleash our thoughts and emotions, which generally sit backstage when our mind is inundated with a flow of continuous stimulation.

Back quite a few decades, when I was growing up, part of waking up involved quietly enjoying the stillness of the morning, allowing my mind to reflect on my dreams while I gradually adjusted to the newness of the day. If I didn't have to get up for school, I would lay there for a while until I fully disengaged from the trance-like state, allowing my mind to gradually resurface. Once alert, I would make my way to the kitchen for breakfast and maybe glance at the newspaper if a parent or sibling hadn't already confiscated it, otherwise, I would read what was on the cereal box. We didn't have alarm clocks, so on a school day our wake-up call would come from the sounds of my father struggling to open the wonky door leading to my bedroom, accompanied by the words, 'Here's a cuppa tea love.'

With that in hand, I would merge into a propped-up position to slowly devour my hot beverage, the spoonful of sugar in the tea alerting my brain from the fogginess of sleep. I would be hypersensitive to the sounds of dad shuffling back to the kitchen and once there, pouring another cuppa for the next sibling in line. The tinkling sound of the sugar being stirred into the tea is still vividly etched in my memory, as the same comforting routine repeated itself over during my childhood years. The few minutes I remained in bed to finish my beverage allowed my mind total peace and quiet from the new day's forthcoming events.

Today, I am a few decades into my adult years and, as the world has changed, so have my habits. Now, when I wake and I don't have to get up for work, I will bring a cup of tea back to bed, but instead of lying there enjoying the quiet stillness of the morning, allowing my brain to do wake up stretches, I demand that it immediately readjust and fire up all neurons. I have several devices in my bedroom. First, I will pick up the phone to check the time and, whilst I am there, I might quickly peruse Facebook and emails, then I will turn on the television to watch something while I drink my tea. There is usually a book by my bed but my brain has become so accustomed to the instant gratification the screens provide, that it has become a slow read.

My night routine is similar. I might intend to have an early night, however, that takes a back seat when there's instant entertainment to be had. My intentions are good but once I am indulged in the screen, two hours can slip by very quickly. First, it's a game on my phone to help me unwind; intended time, 10 minutes; actual time, at least 30 minutes (I'm already embarrassed). Next, I might check social media (who needs to purchase magazines anymore?), then check for any new emails (it's always exciting to see what's in your letterbox, right?) and then, if I haven't used up too much time I will "chillax" with Netflix. Even if I have spent more time than intended, my brain is wired and melatonin suppressed with all the blue light consumption, that I allow more time for all of these addictive activities, forgetting the significance of respite required by the brain to slow down body functions, necessary to drift into sleep mode. Not to mention all this online activity exposing me to increased electromagnetic frequencies. Cross fingers my salt lamp helps neutralise some of those.

I am in the process of gradually changing my habits. Good intentions don't always prevail. At least one night a week I ditch all screens in favour of reading a hand-held book. I'm not too good at it yet. I used to live in a time when a good novel was a luxury and remember how, when reading before sleep, my eyelids would flicker just when I was up to a really good part of the story. I would then have to reluctantly put the book aside or, had I persevered, find the book had dropped from my hands as sleep prevailed. I have never, as yet, fallen asleep to later find my mobile device slipped from my clutches. If ever I am aware of feeling sleepy, I can easily suppress the gateway to natural changes in brain wave frequencies, by simply switching apps.

I remember a time when reading a book was considered a healthy activity to help relax the mind before sleep. Technical devices, apart from a radio, weren't a part of the bedroom setting. The only screen lived in the lounge room, so books were often taken to the bedroom for a nighttime read. Now, I find it a battle to disengage from the addictiveness of instant gratification that our personal devices provide us. With the multitude of options technology presents and its addictive nature, it is easy to succumb to the power it has over us. And when we are spellbound, the true source of our awareness, of all we think and feel, remains somewhere backstage making fleeting appearances here and there. It is easy to forget that we need to draw the curtains, clear the stage, take a break and allow our unencumbered mind to take lead performance.

In a world of digital technology, we have become complacent in taking good care of our minds. Constant incoming stimuli from digital devices and the mentality of filling in every spare moment is detrimental to both our mental and physical wellbeing. The brain needs spontaneous quiet time to internalise and evaluate information. It is too difficult to process thoughts, concentrate on a task, tap into memory and problem solve when we are inundated with external distractions.

Take reading a book for instance. You can ponder over paragraphs, flip back and forth through pages and even avert your eyes to indulge in a period of daydreaming. The only interruptions that disrupt the flow, come from the thoughts roaming around in your head, as opposed to ads and messages constantly interrupting text online. Imagination is allowed to run free. There is no flitting from several sources of information, suppressing your thoughts. Instead, the mind's gateway is open and receptive to be able to absorb and decipher material input from just the one source. Take a moment to consider the difference in spending 30 minutes surfing social media, as opposed to 30 minutes indulging in a good piece of literature.

Constant periods of noise can cause stress and tension as it activates the sympathetic drive of the central nervous system stimulating adrenaline production and heightening alertness. We need periods of silence to gain mental clarity, to exercise imagination, to rest and reflect and to slow down body functions. We need to obtain a harmonious state to reset and regulate all systems on a cellular level. When in idle mode, the brain can make preparations for sleep by switching off the neocortex and secreting hormones necessary for sleep to occur. Sufficient melatonin needs to be released, not only to initiate sleep, but to maintain good quality sleep. It is a known fact that artificial light, as well as other stimulants, suppress melatonin production. We are now privy to a smorgasbord of options bypassing the natural tendency to wind down before sleep. Instead, we can remain hot-wired well into the night.

Working or playing well after sundown may seem conducive to getting more done and having more time, but it comes at a price. It means forfeiting sleep time, which is, in effect, counterproductive, as the extended hours spent achieving more, will eventually have to be made up in rest if the brain is expected to work at full capacity. Extended wake time subtracts from required sleep time. The mind just won't function as efficiently if it is sleep deprived.

We have created a society of wanting more hours in the day as we don't think we have enough. Once there was a time when day and night were evenly divided. Now, we can draw up our own timelines, these being assisted if we live in one of the 70 countries worldwide that practice daylight savings. Switching off from a busy world is difficult, particularly when more hours are dedicated to productivity. Lengthening days by providing more daylight hours can lull us into a false sense of security of having more time to play with.

How much do we really switch off from the world during our time out? Often our leisure time incorporates the use of technology. Even though we may feel as though we are switching off, our brains are still very much in work mode. To totally disconnect, we should free ourselves of all outside disturbances, including digital devices to give the mind total reprieve, absolute quiet.

Total reprieve taps into our intuitive abilities which enhances our creativity and performance. It is often only in the stillness of our mind that we are open to perceptive insights. When our mind is otherwise preoccupied, intuition sits in the background unable to find a way forth and, when it does try to make an appearance, other mind occupants push it backward.

You don't need to be on a desert island swinging on a hammock between coconut trees. However, that would be very nice indeed. Whether you are on a vacation or staycation or simply have a few moments to yourself, indulge in some pure nothingness. Mind bliss.

THE POWER OF NO

Time management is congruent with the ability of being able to say no. Our time is precious and we don't need to flit any of it away on things that are unimportant to us. No frees up space; it buys us time. Whenever we say yes to things, we sacrifice some of our valued time. Sometimes a yes response is well worth the investment and, other times, a no response would really have been the preferred substitute. No is a very essential part of our vocabulary to be able to secure adequate time for our own commitments. The word yes is considered positive and tends to slide out of our mouths quite readily, even before we have had time to contemplate its implications, whereas no resides somewhere in the back alleys, somewhat shy and reserved. It can be a word that can be reckoned with and so, we are hesitant in its use. Even though no is often a preferred or honest response, it is not as fluent as yes and will sometimes need an encouraging nudge.

From a very young age, we have been conditioned to please. No was an off-limit word while yes got all the glory. Yes, was the polite thing to say and as children, we did as our elders taught us. We predominately said yes. Our hands were tied. Adults made the decisions for us and so we were disempowered to say no to anything. If we did say no, it would have been deemed rude and may have gotten us into trouble. As adults, with this kind of background conditioning, it is difficult to associate the no word as something that could be positive. Mature enough to make our own decisions, it is still embedded in us that yes is better than no and so, when we respond to a request, the "nice" word more often comes up trumps.

Requests come in from all over: family, friends, work colleagues, acquaintances and neighbours. Before we know it, we have accepted invitations, meetings and other commitments without giving much thought to how much we may be withdrawing from our time bank. If someone needs our help, we are inclined to give it. Most of us have been brought up with virtues including "love thy neighbour" and so we believe in being a good Samaritan, by giving to others, particularly those in need. We also want to be liked and accepted and not thought badly of and we soon discover that yes earns us brownie points whereas no disappoints. Merrily travelling along the righteous path of being kind, helpful and thoughtful and putting others needs before our own, we sometimes end up being pushed over.

I have always admired people who can say no to something or someone that siphons their time. Most of my life I have been a people pleaser and would always give of my time, when sometimes, inside I would feel resentful and annoyed. Time and experience have taught me to pull back the reins somewhat and regain time for the most important things in my life. My priorities come first. I consider myself to be a generous person and I am impartial to giving my time to those who will benefit from my goodwill. Because ultimately, I get something in return. Gratitude. A sense of inner warmth and satisfaction. So, that is well worth my time. However, as you know, there are those people who may take you for granted, use up more of your time than you were prepared to give, or siphon your energy levels, leaving you feeling depleted. This is where I have learned to pull back. As I can't always avoid these people, I can be selective of the time I give them. I have learned through experience, as I am sure so too have you, what saying yes can drag you through.

Saying no to things that don't benefit you or subtracts from your valuable energy, frees up time for what matters to you. Time is priceless and segments of it can be irreplaceable by too many yeses. Saying no can feel uncomfortable, especially if you feel that you are going to disappoint someone, appear rude or mean, or fear people will drop off your friendship list. Why is it that other people can say no with ease and are unscathed by it? It's all to do with confidence. There is a way of delivering the verdict. It has to do with being direct, yet polite. It doesn't involve stumbling over a request with excuses or taking time to think about it. It requires a firm and sincere no. I was always the sucker that extended my shifts or took on extra workloads when others around me were getting off scot-free. Sure, maybe I was admired for this but I was also easy prey, which only led to frustration and envy and less me time. The more you give, the more people learn to take and the more you stand out as an easy target.

Be aware that saying yes doesn't always gain respect and consideration from recipients as it perhaps should. Sometimes you may give of your time to help someone with a workload, a project or favour, or you may nominate a listening ear to their troubles. You were taught to put others needs before your own and so you willingly go out of your way to assist. Your time is sacrificed in doing a good deed for another. It is rewarding to be able to help someone and sometimes a 'thank you' in return is all you need. Beware of the time consumables; people that take more than they ever give back. We all know of these people, right? It is important to set boundaries as sometimes they can be leeches, draining your time and energy numerous times over. Make your yeses count; you should get something in return: a sense of achievement, enjoyment or satisfaction in helping someone. Sacrificing time and energy has to mean something to you.

How many of us have expected a returned favour that hasn't been forthcoming? Sometimes we do more for another than they ever do for us. Accept that. That's the way it is. Decipher who these people are in your life and, where possible, pull back from them. It may be difficult to avoid doing more than your fair share, especially if you are dealing with family members or close friends. Know that these people may not give you a fair trade but there will be others in your life that are more giving and so, accept this as a gift from the universe, to make up for the unfairness. As infuriating as it is, you may get burnt by some, yet there will be others who will dress your wounds.

When you find it difficult to say no, think of the consequences of saying yes. If a yes response puts a dampener on your mood, causes resentment or takes you away from how you wanted to spend your time, then the benefits of no will far outweigh the discomfort of a yes response. The aftermath of yes can cause unwarranted stress. This stress can hang around for a longer than anticipated time, shattering your equilibrium. Something as simple as the nuisance phone call can be enough to cause upset. You don't recognise the number but you pick up anyway. There is a delay, indicating that you could probably just hang up straight away as it is just as you expect: some telemarketer offering a product or service you're not the least bit interested in. But you have held on. A voice presents, usually in a heavy accent, and talking at a phenomenal speed to get as much information across whilst you are still listening. Already wishing you had hung up, you now feel obliged to listen for what is considered a polite amount of time before disclosing your disinterest. At some point you hang up. How has it made you feel? Most likely annoyed for having silently said yes by accepting the call. You may have been intrigued at first but hung on longer than intended or sorry that you didn't just hang up right at the beginning of the call. After all, their aim is to persuade and manipulate you into saying yes. You know this, which only accentuates the regret of taking the bait. Whether for just a few moments or longer, the salesperson stole time from you. Time you weren't willingly prepared to give away, especially to a stranger. There are numerous other examples of readily giving away yes and your reaction will be determined by the situation and how much time it costs you. Your resentment could last several minutes, hours or days. Worst case scenario, it may find a permanent residence in your subconscious, making fleeting appearances and dampening your mood from time to time.

There are times when a yes feels like the appropriate response in the context of acceptances to parties, weddings or other social events. But in reality, these things cut into your time or invitations come from those who are not on your "close people" list. Saying no in these incidents can be tricky. Maybe you have limited time but you don't want to say no for fear of missing out on something good or, maybe you don't want to decline an invitation because the host values your presence. Yes, then comes from a place of not wanting to disappoint or hurt someone. Yet you do have yourself to think about and the consequences of the yes response. You have to ask yourself, how important is it to you when it involves shedding another layer of your valuable time?

No is often challenged. Yes, on the other hand is readily accepted and, on the surface, gains you popularity. It often seems an easier response than no. Ultimately, a yes response presents no conflict. A no response can open up a debate. People will often press you to justify yourself. This can feel uncomfortable and disclose more than you wish to reveal. Holding your ground by standing firm will gain you more respect in the long run than multiple yeses will. Eventually, you may lose respect if you cave in too easily to yes. You may be deemed submissive and taken advantage of. Besides, it is difficult to form trust in people who are always agreeable.

There are things we need to say no to, so that we can give wholly of ourselves. We can't jam pack everything into one day or weekend, allowing small snippets of time to relationships and think that a bit of time is better than none. Relationships require nurturing and so, it is better to structure time around things that really matter, giving less time to things that don't.

Mobile devices can interrupt quality time spent with others. Unless you are expecting an important call or message, it is best to leave the mobile phone in your pocket or bag when engaged in a social setting. Preferably turned off. It is disconcerting when someone in the company of others, constantly diverts their eyes to the phone sitting on the table, worse still, when they engage in its presence.

In a society where time is becoming more and more precious, much of it can be wasted submerged in a virtual reality. A simple gesture of checking the time on a technical device can easily lead to opening up notifications and, before long, being swept into an oblivion, unaware of the passage of time. Emerging from the trance, with the intention of viewing the time, which your brain was initially too distracted to properly register, you refresh your look and note that what seemed like a few minutes is so much more. You inadvertently bumped up the setting on your life treadmill and feel cheated. Perhaps it would have been better to have glanced at a wall clock or wristwatch that isn't a smart device. No often involves self-restraint and discipline.

Our internal impulses constantly need addressing. Managing our priorities often involves containing our urges. We know what the better deal is but we have continual battles with the yes/no voices in our head. Yes, is the loudest and quickest to respond, with no, trailing behind somewhere in the distance. You may start out with the best intentions only to discover you have succumbed to the first response. Feeling disappointed in your lack of restraint and, as you have already slipped into the rabbit hole, you may risk losing all self-control and allow yourself to free fall in. With our minds swaying us in two different directions, we need to discipline ourselves in making the right choices beneficial to our wellbeing. Just as empowering as it is to say no to others, so too is it when it involves making wise decisions for ourselves.

Time matters. Time is limited. You own the time you have, so be selective in giving it away or utilising it in a manner you aren't comfortable with. Say no to things or commitments if they cause frustration, resentment or hurt. Saying no opens up more time to accomplish your personal goals, relax and enjoy time spent on activities and the people who are most important to you. Allow the possibilities of what you could say yes to, inspire your no response.

When you say yes, set boundaries so your energy remains at a healthy level. Our bodies need to be in sync on all levels: physical, emotional and spiritual, otherwise something will begin to give way and we cannot function at our ultimate best. We may get stuck, become undone and let negative and abusive people seep into our lives.

Keep time for important relationships in your life. Don't sit under the mat of being walked over by those who take advantage of you. Make more profound and loving connections with people of the same frequency as you, to maintain harmony and balance in your life. There are many demands on your personal time in this life. You have your own agenda to which you need to allocate time. Make that your priority and be discriminative to who or what you give any other time to. When no seems a rude or uncomfortable response, consider your mental health and sanity.

EXCUSITIS

People can fall into being complacent in their lives. They live in a comfortable bubble forgoing the opportunity and chance cards. Just playing life by the rules to keep on even keel and avoid risk taking. This may seem like the safest option in the game, as there are less hurdles to jump, which equates to less falls. With this style of game playing, the forward moves are limited; there are no detours or unexpected surprises. Setbacks are few, as the field of vision is narrowed with peripheral vision switched off. The way through the game is tentative, as situations causing any diversion need to be avoided. The disadvantage of this game style is that the game cannot be played to its full potential. Optional moves are obstructed as they involve exercising risk.

There are many forms of excusitis: excuses we make for non-achievements and staying stuck. I am sure you've heard them all: I was never given the opportunity; I came from a dysfunctional or poor family; I am not smart or young enough; I haven't got the time. What's really being said is: I'm afraid of failure; I don't want to face my fears; I don't want to make a spectacle of myself; I'm not good enough. You could say that excusitis protects us from failure. Failure can carry the consequences of disappointment and embarrassment. So, if you plod along in life, avoiding opportunities that potentially subject you to risk, you will certainly be playing it safe. However, in doing so, you will forfeit living life to the fullest and exercising your unique talents.

Talent can lie dormant if not exercised. Recognising opportunities, accepting challenges and performing at your best can bring out hidden abilities. Fear can block your natural flair, talent that you may never know exists unless it's awakened by accepting challenges. It is easy to attribute success to good luck and lack of success to bad luck. This attitude assumes things just happen in life for some people as they are lucky to be born with exceptional talents or, conversely, bad luck just follows some people around and, unfortunately, that's just the way it is. But is it really? If we take a close look into the lives of successful people, we would see just how much effort they put into their successes and how many knock-backs/failures these, so called, achievers had before they made it. The bottom line, with anyone who is successful, is they never give up trying. Even if they don't ever quite achieve what they set out to do, they don't quit and so they gather a repertoire of lessons along the way which, in itself, is a great accomplishment. People who try and then give up because it didn't work out the first or second time, don't have the advantage of these lessons that can be applied to so many aspects of life.

Excuses can become a burden to haul throughout life. Taking action dissolves the burden. You will feel better for having taken action, rather than packing another 'can't do it' into your luggage to cart around. Doing lightens your load and enables growth. Think about how good you feel after you've taken initiative. Every time you put something off, it's an added weight to lug around. Often enough, the desire is present but the action required to get there is lagging. Something may be attempted with all good intention but left unfinished because of a lack of motivation or because the task becomes too challenging.

Procrastination is something we all go through from time to time. Often, tiredness can make us lazy and unmotivated and so we put something off, picking it up at another time when we are well rested. That's normal. That's human. That's allowed. Once we feel up to it, ticking things off on our to-do-list can be divided into urgent and non-urgent. What is essential to get done right now and what isn't? Know what you need to give immediate attention to and what can wait. Things that are unimportant can have less time allocated to them or even be eliminated from the list if they get in the way of more essential tasks. Beware that procrastination can tempt you to spend more time on the easy things on your list, that don't require the time or attention than the more difficult tasks require. Confront the temptation to procrastinate and tackle the most arduous and anxiety provoking task to get it done. If you are worried about the tension and effort it will take, think of how good you will feel once it is achieved. You could promise yourself a treat after its completion if that helps you get motivated.

Negative thinking is a precursor of procrastination. It is preferable to delay something through fear of making a mistake or appearing like a failure. We can hold back because we don't think we have the required talent or worry about what others may think or, because the task is too time-consuming, requiring too much effort. The more you procrastinate, the more negative you feel. You could end up not doing anything, then start to feel guilty for not trying. Feelings of self-doubt and helplessness start to seep in, overriding all intentions and you end up stuck.

Sometime along the life path, you may have been conditioned to believe there are certain things you cannot achieve and you come to accept this. You may brave giving it a go and, if it doesn't work out the first time, insecurities, self-doubts and hesitation all get in the way of trying again. You limit your attempts as, that way, you are staying safe and not inviting risk. The way around this is to change your mode of thinking. It is all in the way we train our thoughts. Success stories come from positive thinking. Negative thinking limits opportunities and paralyses creativity. Develop the appropriate mindset.

It is all too easy to set aside something for another time and fill in the space with some other activity so as not to address the issue. "Not having the time" excuses really translate into not having the inclination. Sometimes, we are all guilty of shoving things in the too hard basket and leaving them there to be unaddressed indefinitely. Deep down, we know we will never pull those items out of our basket, but we kid ourselves into thinking that one day we will. That one day will only ever happen if we change our thought processes.

There are tasks, opportunities and events in life that require effort and brain power. Unless we put in these elements, we won't reap all that life has to offer us. Success comes in many forms. You don't need to be smart enough or have a high IQ to be successful. All that is required is a thinking brain and, once that thinking brain is switched on, it needs to be allowed to go where it will, unhindered by time or inhibitions that could easily shut it down. Use your mind to create and develop ideas. You can open your mind to succeed. It is not a matter of good luck for some. Success takes planning and hard work and if you fail, take the fall, so be it. The most successful people have had numerous tumbles. It's about picking yourself back up and getting straight back on the bucking bull again. Take the lesson you have learned from the failure and apply it to your next attempt. If the bull keeps tossing you off, at least you can be satisfied that you have given it a fair go and can then move onto something else.

Failure can be considered an opportunity of re-evaluating goals. In dissecting the situation, we will discover the qualities and skills we have and those which we need to acquire or develop. Failure can shed light on pathways we need to take to improve our efficiency. Don't expect perfection. Just putting in the effort of trying and not being put off by failure is good enough. When it all seems too hard and discouragement extinguishes action, look back on past achievements and consider the effort you had put in and the contentment you felt when a project came to fruition.

Success is rewarding. Once something is accomplished, there's no more procrastinating over it. There is an exhilaration at the end of achieving a task, particularly if it has required considerable effort. The natural high obtained drives enthusiasm and excitement to achieve more, take on other quests and be further challenged. People confined to their bubble don't see the rich harvest of opportunities available to them. They are resistant to change and don't go out of their way looking for opportunities or challenges. They go on living their lives carrying around disappointment because they don't take the necessary steps to make change. This becomes burdensome and has the propensity to lead to anxiety and fear, escalating to the temptation to anaesthetise these feelings with tranquillisers and stimulants, rather than face the fact they are stagnant or in the wrong place.

Successful people stand out from the crowd. They are

seen to be doers which gains them popularity and trust. Their reliability assures them passage of moving up the ranks in their fields as they take on more responsibility and more important tasks. Devoid of excuses, they confront challenges head on, powering through them, despite the efforts and struggles experienced.

Being human, we all slip into a lazy or "can't be bothered" mode from time to time. We could be legitimately too tired, sick or depressed to muster up the energy to achieve goals, take on a new project, accept an invitation or just complete tasks. We are allowed this time out in life. In fact, this reprieve can refresh and empower us, enabling us the energy and motivation to perform at our best at a more suitable time.

It doesn't matter where we are in life, how young we are or how old. We are alive and still in the game, so unless illness or debilitation limits us, what we make of our lives is up to us. We have the tools and resources to create our desired existence. Each of us will have our own specific preferences. Success comes in small, medium and large packages. What we need to remember is that through desire, goal setting and determined effort, along with persistence, success will be achievable in one form or another. Even the smallest of successes counts.

Throughout our lives we are constantly presented with opportunities. The more opportunities we accept, the more lessons we learn. We have a choice. Sometimes we go out on a limb accepting challenges that are risky or that may involve criticism from other people but we forge ahead anyway. Sometimes we succeed and sometimes we fail. The bigger the challenge, the bigger the learning curve. You can learn just as much if not more from failure as you can from success. Partaking in these lessons that life provides us, enables personal growth which is a process of trial, error and experimentation.

Don't be afraid of failure. Take a chance. If you choose an opportunity card that seems out of reach, break it down into small pieces and, as you work toward attaining your goal, you may just notice yourself growing and expanding, surprised at being so absorbed in the project. If you fall, get up again and have another go or try something else. Mistakes are progress; they are lessons learned. Concentrate on the positives. If it is a task that won't be repeated, take what you have gained from it. Be willing to always stretch your comfort zone. Even when you don't attain the goals you set out to, you will reap the rewards of emotional and intellectual growth.

If we choose to forgo many of the opportunities available to us, we opt for a more mediocre life. We may kid ourselves and pocket opportunities for another time. Ten, 20, 30 years go by so quickly. Some opportunities in life won't present again. We can't hold back time or think we have plenty ahead of us. If we want something, we have to strike while the iron is hot and not get lost in the pretence of later. Time is ticking.

PART FOUR

Choice Cards

WHAT IS GOOD ENOUGH

We are a human species, assigned to planet earth to play out our lives. In this life, we have been given a stock of resources to use for our benefit. We draw upon these resources to better our existence. There are many decisions to be made on which resources to use and these decisions will reflect what we consider to be good enough.

We have been issued many choice cards with which we can do as we please. There was a time before we became independent, a time before being fully released into the playground of life, that these choice cards were selected by our parents and caregivers. Decisions were made for us, based on the cards chosen. Sometimes, these choices made on our behalf, all in goodwill, weren't always the right ones. Our parents and carers didn't have a guidance manual and so they sometimes fumbled in choosing the right cards. Decisions made were influenced by their own upbringing, knowledge and experiences.

Once we become independent members of society, all cards are laid out on the table for our own choosing and we become solely responsible for making our own decisions affecting our livelihood. Again, as with those preceding us, these decisions are under the influence of our knowledge or lack thereof, experiences we have previously encountered and the manner in which we have been raised. Our free will and ignorance sometimes get in the way of selecting the right cards.

We are each given a body to exist in. We may like it or not, but it is ours for keeps for as long as we live. This is the temple of our being. How we take care of it will determine our quality of life, which will, in effect, have an enormous influence on our general wellbeing and longevity. Our temple consists of body, mind and soul, all of which require an equal amount of servicing. Choices are consistently made to tweak this servicing and, ideally, all three constituents should be synchronised to create a harmonious balance.

There are many areas in our life in which we have to make choices. Choices that are good enough to get us around the game board and through all levels. Decisions made aren't always easy or necessarily the right ones. It is natural to expect setbacks as some of our choices backfire. That is just the realism of being human. It is also a vital part of our learning experience. Life is full of lessons. We don't just learn them all in a set amount of time. Lessons continue from the moment of birth until the moment of death. And even then, when life wraps up and the game is over, there are most likely to be lessons missed.

Imagine being back at school, concentrating in class on every single lesson. By the end of the day, would you be able to recall all that you had learned? Probably not. Sometimes it would have been difficult to recall much at all, depending on your attention span at the time. Most likely, you would have been issued some homework or study; to further embed the learned information so it could be retained for later recall. Then there would be some sort of test, an exam or assignment and so you would have to set aside some time to focus on the subject through study and research. It would be impossible otherwise, to cram everything in all at once, as without some sort of concentrated focus on the subject, the brain just doesn't have the capacity to retain everything in detail.

In life, we learn new things through our experiences and if we were to be tested on what we had learned through these experiences, our score would depend on how present we were at the time. There are many obstacles that may hinder the uptake of the lesson besides concentration span. Self-worth, self-awareness, values and beliefs, the state of our physical health and our emotional status all contribute to how engaged we are in the experience. Sometimes we simply miss the lesson of the experience altogether because we are closed-off to it.

Throughout life, we grow and mature. Our values and beliefs may change according to our experiences. We can also feel differently about ourselves during various stages of our life cycle. As knowledge accumulates, attitudes change, life experiences, although similar or the same to what we have previously encountered, may be viewed from a different perspective. And so, we continue to learn something new, something else, not only from new experiences but also from those that are repeated.

Even when we have learned something and gathered the goods from the learning experience, the lesson sometimes falls out of our memory bank. We either forget it or we stash it somewhere deep in our files and can't retrieve it. Other experiences come in, looking for a spare filing cabinet, making it difficult to hold onto all that we have committed to memory. Some of it just needs to be pushed aside.

Oliver Hardt, a research psychologist who studies memory and forgetting states, 'Without forgetting, we would have no memory at all. If we remembered everything, we would be completely inefficient because our brains would be swamped with superfluous memories.' He goes on to explain that the brain doesn't instantly know what is and isn't important, so it grabs onto everything first, later filtering out the unimportant stuff.

There is a consolidation process that cements an important memory. New information comes in constantly. Some of it is filed in the short-term memory and if it is deemed important it will be transferred to long-term memory. Memories that are most strongly encoded occur when we are paying attention, are deeply engaged and when information is interesting to us. We can be selective in encoding information which explains how one person's recollection of an event may be different to another who shared the exact same experience.

As already established, if the brain had no capacity for memory, information would be lost. There would be no point in learning anything as it wouldn't be retained. To play the life game to the best of our ability, it is preferable to have an accessible collection of memories in our long-term memory bank. The more packed our reference files are with accumulated information we have learned or experienced, the more equipped we are to play the various levels of the game. And what better way is there than to surrender our full attention to life's moments, to expand our memory bank?

In order to get the most out of life, we need to be functioning to the best of our capacity. And that requires keeping our health in check. A nutritious diet, sufficient sleep and exercise all contribute to an optimal functioning body. We need to get it right, where it counts and that is, on a cellular level. It all starts in the mitochondria, which are housed in each of our trillions of cells. The mitochondria are the energy store houses in each of our body's cells. They are responsible for producing the energy our bodies require to function. We need to fuel these little tackers so they can convert substances from the foods we eat into energy. Adenosine triphosphate (ATP) is the energy generated from our cell's mitochondria and is used to facilitate all of our biochemical and physiological processes responsible for maintaining our body's homeostasis.

As well as the food we eat, the air we breathe is vital in maintaining healthy mitochondrial function. The bloodstream picks up oxygen from the lungs and transports it into the cells where it is used for cellular energy production. Carbon dioxide, a waste product of this process, is then delivered back to the lungs where it can be excreted from the body. Mitochondria are responsible for performing house cleaning duties throughout the body, from mopping up damaged cells to regenerating new ones and regulating our innate immune system. The more energised the mitochondria are, the better this service is. Exercise delivers more oxygen to all of our body's cells, stimulating mitochondrial biogenesis. So, the more we move, the more our cells produce these energy power packs keeping our bodies in pristine working condition.

Sleep is also an important factor in mitochondrial function, keeping our bodies in tip top shape. Poor quality and quantity of sleep can affect immune function as well as the body's ability to heal and repair. Some of our cells need to be restored to optimal function and others need to be eliminated from the body, most of which occurs during sleep. Insufficient sleep can lead to oxidative stress where there is an imbalance between free radicals and antioxidants in the body. Free radicals, unstable atoms that cause damage to cells, are generated consistently in the body and antioxidants, which are neutralising compounds, are required to engulf these menacing irritants. Antioxidants need to swamp these free radicals to keep our bodies balanced and ward off premature ageing and disease.

Healthy mitochondrial function depends on how we treat our bodies. Everyday decisions on what we eat, how much we move/exercise and how much time we devote to rest and sleep are imperative in keeping us in homeostasis. If the core energy units of our cells are disabled, all bodily systems are affected, impacting our overall wellbeing.

Our physical and mental health needs to be good enough to be able to concentrate on other components of our lives. According to The World Health Organization (WHO), health is defined as a state of complete physical, mental and social wellbeing. There is a core relationship between physical and mental health; a mind-body connection which makes it impossible for one to exist without the other. If we are physically fit, we are more readily able to keep our emotional health in check and vice versa. Chronic physical disease will have an impact on mental wellness and poor mental health can be a catalyst for deteriorating physical health.

Living a good enough life means different things for different people, but we all have a common denominator, which involves living a life beyond the means of just survival. I think it would be fair to say we all strive for the best in life, for both ourselves and our loved ones. To maximise our existence, it is important to feel connected to life and to achieve this, we need to maintain a reasonably healthy state, both physically and mentally. As much as we need our senses to navigate the world, in order to function optimally, these need to be partnered with our mental faculties. We need to take the time to nurture and respect our body in its entirety, so we can fully immerse ourselves in life as it happens. The healthier we are, the wider our spectrum of life and the more equipped we are to deal with whatever life throws our way.

Life is mysterious and has the uncanny ability of surprising us every day. Sometimes, life happens as we expect it to and sometimes it doesn't. We can be caught off guard at any moment. What we may think of as a routine ordinary type of day, can suddenly take a turn on us to become something more complex. The unexpected event, news, diagnosis, accident or whatever else, may completely throw us off kilter. Bamboozled by an abrupt change in events, we can find ourselves frantically grappling for a survival kit, in the hope of finding something appropriate to use for the whirlwind of emotions and panic that suddenly trespassed our state of equilibrium. The game has changed and we are expected to play a different hand. One of which we had most unlikely prepared for. We do the best we can to change tactics in the hope of finding a way back to a harmonious state. No one welcomes these diversions in life but they are necessary to broaden our perspectives and, ultimately, open up opportunities for personal growth. The hurdles, the tumbles and the cracks in the path alert us to delve deeper into our inner wisdom. There is so much knowledge in what we have learned and stored in our memory bank awaiting our retrieval. There is also new information to collect, to be stored as newfound knowledge. Wherever life turns, there is always something to be gained and our adaptation to any new circumstance will reflect our state of wellbeing.

COMPONENTS OF HEALTH

To stretch out our time on earth and to live a healthy life, we know we have to take particular care of our travelling vessels. The body we were issued needs to be nurtured to generate optimal performance. That means keeping our physical, mental and spiritual wellbeing in check. Nutrition, exercise and sleep are all important in keeping us in good shape. You can't maintain health on a good diet and skimp on sleep, just as you can't eat and sleep well and not bother with exercise. We need to eat. We need to move. We need to sleep.

Our choices count. They shape our life. Let's begin with diet, exercise and sleep. We all know that if we eat well, exercise regularly and sleep sufficient hours, we will be boarding the healthy life carriage. This is a rickety carriage to remain on throughout life's entirety. And most of us have to reboard it numerous times along the journey. There are times in our lives when we select easier or more pleasurable carriages that forfeit good habits. Who hasn't ever indulged in unhealthy food options or mind-altering substances, chosen a day of complete idleness or elected to stay up all night to party on? Of course, we all have choices and to do something off rail can feel quite exhilarating and break the boredom that can be associated with rigid clean living.

Diet, exercise and sleep are inextricably linked. It is all about balance. Food provides fuel for exercise. Exercise helps distribute oxygen and nutrients to our cells and prepares the body's biochemistry for a good night's sleep. And when we have good quality sleep, we are more likely to make healthier food choices and be motivated to exercise. And on it goes.

We have an abundance of knowledge at our fingertips regarding healthy food choices. We know we should mostly eat healthy, wholesome foods, preferably void of pesticides, additives and preservatives. Our lifestyle has far surpassed that of our hunter and gatherer ancestors and we have a wide option of food choices available to us, which makes it more difficult to be restrictive and stick to the untampered foods of the land. Dietary guidelines are always changing but we do know it is best to consume a diet predominantly rich in plant foods and limit fats, carbohydrates and added sugar. We live in an era of convenience foods which are usually easy, pleasing to the palate, and require little, if any, preparation time. These foods suit our busy lifestyles and are easy to grab on the run. Their downside is, they can be laden with additives which may be a deterrent to our overall health. More and more convenience foods are populating the market, making them an easier choice, particularly in time-poor scenarios.

We share our bodies with trillions of microorganisms which help protect us against disease. These organisms make up the microbiome or normal flora of the body. The body's microbiome helps protect our bodies by laying down colonies, making it difficult for disease-causing bacteria to invade. Gut microbiome plays an important role in regulating immune function, aiding the synthesis of important vitamins and assisting digestion. What we put through our digestive tract greatly affects the ecosystem of microbes that live in the gut. A healthy gut microbiome is consistent with eating a balanced diet consisting of a wide variety of plant-based foods, reducing stress and getting regular exercise and sleep. Excessive sugar consumption, antibiotics, surgeries, chemotherapy and heavy metals are some of the things that can confiscate good bacteria and lower intestinal flora.

The immune system is intricately related to gut microbiota and when the two are in harmony, the body is equipped to deal with pathogens keeping it in homeostasis. The gut microbiome teaches the immune cells, known as T-cells, to identify foreign entities and these in coexistence with macrophages get to work to scavenge and eliminate unwelcome intruders. When everything is in order, the gut directs immune cells to attack invading pathogens and, in turn, the immune system helps in keeping the microbiome well populated with healthy microbes. A normal functioning digestive tract requires a diversity of microbiome and anything that alters the composition of microbial populations can lead to chronic inflammation and metabolic dysfunction. The lining of the gut is delicate and when weakened, minute tears can occur in the intestinal wall allowing harmful invaders to permeate through. This is known as leaky bowel syndrome. This can cascade into a host of systemic symptoms and contribute to a wide range of medical conditions. Good health starts with the quality and quantity of the microbiome living on and within us. We need our little army posted on every internal and external surface with a surplus stationed in the barracks.

What are the effects of sugar in our diet and why is it that something that tastes so glorious should only be consumed in moderation? It seems ridiculously unfair. Unfortunately, too much sugar can play havoc on the body. We actually get plenty of sugar through natural sources such as fruit and vegetables, without the need to consume added sugar. Over consumption of sugar can create inflammation, a raised blood sugar level, thickened more viscous blood, leading to high blood pressure, heart disease, obesity and cancer. A high sugar diet can activate the body's immune response which, in effect, can lead to a chronic inflammatory state. This occurs because sugar offsets the production of free fatty acids in the liver and the breakdown of these products triggers inflammatory processes. In a chronic inflammatory state, healthy cells can be attacked and there is less time for body processes to perform housecleaning, leaving damaged cells and toxins to accumulate within the body.

Our bodies release insulin from the pancreas in order to collect sugar deposited into the bloodstream, where it is then transported to the cells and used for energy. Any excess glucose, the simplest form of sugar, is then stored in the muscles, liver and fatty tissue. The intake of sugar causes an immediate spike in blood sugar levels, which activates insulin to deal with the redistribution of glucose into storage.

A diet high in sugar can lead to obesity and subsequent insulin resistance. Insulin resistance occurs when the cells in our storage compartments (muscles, liver and body fat), start to ignore messages of accepting glucose from the bloodstream. As the body stops responding to the hormone insulin, the pancreas goes into overdrive producing more insulin in an attempt to lower blood sugar levels. Eventually there's a full-on wrestle. The demand on the pancreas becomes too much. It can't keep up and the excess sugar in the bloodstream begins to damage blood vessels. The rise in blood sugar can eventually lead to vascular disease, kidney disease, visual disturbances and nerve damage. Interestingly, insulin resistance can also be caused by a lack of exercise and sleep. Movement enables the muscle cells to take up glucose more readily and studies indicate that sleep is essential in maintaining blood sugar levels.

Sugar is a toxin which fuels diabetes, obesity, heart disease and cancer. It accelerates ageing and inflammation in the body. Advanced glycation end products (AGES) are toxic compounds formed by reactions between sugars and proteins in the body. These AGEs accumulate naturally as we age and we have antioxidants and enzymes to mop up these harmful compounds but, when levels become increasingly high, the body can't keep up, leading to oxidative stress and inflammation. This insult on the body will eventually stymie tissue and organ repair consequently leading to disease. AGEs are also known to form when certain foods are cooked at high temperatures. Animal foods that are high in fat and protein are more susceptible to AGE formation during cooking, particularly when cooked quickly and at high heat. A little hint – it is better to choose slow cooking as an alternative method of cooking meat, over roasting, grilling and frying and marinating in acidic ingredients, to reduce AGE production.

Modern diets can contribute to higher levels of AGEs in the body. Natural antioxidants have the ability to neutralise the effects of, as well as accumulation of, AGEs. This is why it is good to include plenty of plant-based foods, including herbs and spices, to counteract any potential tissue damage that could otherwise occur when advanced glycation end products are allowed to accumulate. Interestingly, AGE production is reduced by exercise and quality sleep. Movement helps deliver the necessary antioxidants and enzymes to filter out these waste products and it is during sleep when the body focuses on repair, that toxin elimination occurs.

Fruit and vegetables are full of antioxidants and anti-inflammatory compounds that help reduce the risk of chronic inflammation. As well as sugars, other foods that cause inflammation include refined carbohydrates, trans fat found in fast food and fried food and saturated fats found in red meat and dairy products. Animal products also carry toxins, which can offset an inflammatory response that can last for hours following their ingestion. The more toxins your body has to deal with, the less time it has for repair. It becomes very busy digesting and processing everything that's going into it, with little opportunity to send out rescue cells to other parts of the body that need restoration.

It is so easy to ditch healthier food choices for more convenient foods. After all, they taste great and are quick to satisfy. Many fast foods stimulate the production of dopamine which leaves us craving more. If only there was an instant reward signal activated by our digestive tract when we deposited something good into it. But no, there are no green lights or bells and whistles for that. Our bodies keep silent. We just have to trust that, how we nourish our bodies will be reflected in our health.

Sugar can be considered as addictive as alcohol, tobacco and illicit drugs. This is because it behaves in the same way. Sugar lights up the brain creating an instant dopamine and serotonin release. This creates a pleasant feeling that craves reinforcement. The reward regions of the brain are short lived as sugar is metabolised quickly, leading to a craving of needing the next fix. A pattern establishes. An instant high, followed by an equally swift plummet in feel good hormones, can lead to feelings of anxiety, depression and fatigue which can then lead to a yearning for more of what created that preferred warm, fuzzy, content feeling. Hence, we reach out for more. Simple or refined carbohydrates readily convert to sugar causing that same effect, whereas complex carbohydrates and protein are slower for the body to metabolise with a more gradual release of energy, keeping the body more satisfied and stable. A preferred option compared to the sudden crash and sluggish feeling following sugar withdrawal.

When hungry, our blood sugar levels are low and so we crave sugars and refined carbohydrates for an instant fix. We may overeat, as these foods drive us to eat more and shovel it in faster, leaving little room or inclination for healthier options. Unlike alcohol and drug addiction, sugar doesn't carry the same recognition as an addictive substance, so is often insidious. However, addiction to sugar can have serious long term negative consequences that are as equally detrimental to health. There is an age limit on consumption of alcohol, yet candy/sweets are often introduced at a very young age and, once children mingle in the community, it can't always be patrolled by parents/caregivers.

Exercise helps reduce sugar cravings. As well as being a distraction, exercise boosts endorphin production and, as more blood is being pumped around the body, there is more glucose deposited in the brain. Getting enough sleep is also important in curbing sugar cravings. Leptin is a hormone that helps regulate energy balance. Its key role is to assess energy homeostasis and suppress hunger. Conversely, ghrelin is a hormone that increases appetite. The hypothalamus is directed by these two hormones, telling the brain when to eat and when to stop. A lack of sleep can muddle with the production of these hormones. When the body is tired, leptin secretion is inhibited and ghrelin secretion is increased, which explains why we are hungrier when sleep deprived, usually grabbing foods that are high in calories as they produce instant energy, a quick pick-me-up.

Our bodies are very busy every minute of every day, making new cells, getting rid of dead and damaged cells and eliminating the constant influx of toxins. The replenishment of new cells requires energy and the elimination of old worn-out cells and disease-causing pathogens calls upon the role of our immune system. Digestion requires the expenditure of energy and activates our immune function. Every time we eat, our immune system immediately pounces on what needs to be eliminated from the body and insulin production is turned on, in readiness to transport blood glucose. With the body actively mopping up and sorting out where to deposit the glucose, processes that help eliminate damaged cells wait their turn. These damaged cells are then left to accumulate until the body has a spare moment to deal with them. If the body is kept occupied with digestion, these damaged cells are slower to eliminate which makes the body more vulnerable to disease.

Immune function starts with a healthy gut microbiome to neutralise and filter out harmful invaders. The more diverse your microbiome, the better your immune function. Intermittent fasting gives the body more time for essential repair work. The process of digestion can take six to eight hours. If the body is constantly digesting and eliminating toxins from foods, there is little time for other immune duties. When there is a decent interval between meals, the body is allowed time to perform a spring clean, tidy up old cells, re-energise mitochondria and reboot the diversity of the microbiome. Ideally, if you stop eating after an early dinner and recommence eating the next day at breakfast or brunch, you will find you have fasted for 13 or more hours. Stretching it out a little more than this every so often will boost the benefits.

The food we consume has a direct impact on our health. Nature has it all sorted. Whatever foods come from nature have anti-inflammatory, antioxidant, antibacterial and antifungal properties, protecting gut bacteria and reducing oxidative stress in cells. If we can remember to choose plant-based foods over man-made foods the majority of the time, we will reduce our risk of disease and slow down the ageing process. There's another benefit. In choosing to eat foods of the land, we can reach a comfortable level of satiety without feeling compelled to overeat. This will improve our inclination to exercise as well as our quality of sleep.

Research now shows that regular exercise throughout the day is essential to longevity. Smaller bouts of frequent exercise prove more beneficial than longer bouts of irregular exercise. Moving around every hour or so, engaging in something that moves the body, is better for you than hours of being sedentary with occasional routine boosts of 30-40 minutes of exercise slotted into just one part of the day, no matter how strenuous it may be. Moving, to some extent, every half an hour is most beneficial. Gentle yoga is a great option that can be practiced in smaller time frames with the benefit of reducing stress. The mind-body connection associated with yoga, has the potential of changing the body's biochemistry, reducing inflammatory reactions, thus normalising blood pressure and reducing oxidative stress. There's also the advantage of increasing blood flow and strengthening connective tissue, keeping the body in good alignment.

Exercise has a range of benefits. It improves metabolic and cardiovascular function. Exercise boosts muscle strength, helps maintain a healthy weight, improves mood and promotes better sleep. We need to move to keep our bodies in good working order. Our heart pumps blood around the body and it does so more efficiently when we exercise. When we move, our heart rate increases which improves circulation. More blood flow enables more oxygen to be delivered to our cells which, in turn, permits the uptake of waste products from cellular activity back into the bloodstream to be eliminated from the body. As blood is pumped around the body at a faster rate during exercise as opposed to when we are idle, our metabolic rate also increases which helps regulate energy levels. Blood glucose is redirected into cells for immediate use or deposited into the liver and muscles for storage. An increase in circulating blood volume improves brain perfusion, increasing the uptake of oxygen and nutrients and promoting brain plasticity by stimulating growth of new connections between cells. Well oxygenated brain cells enhance cognitive skills, memory, performance and retrieval of stored information. Aerobic exercise such as walking, gardening, swimming, cycling or jogging can be protective of the hippocampus (a brain structure that is responsible for learning and memory) which naturally shrinks as we age. Exercise could well be a contributing factor in maintaining a sharp mind in old age.

Endocannabinoids are molecules made by the body which help keep our internal functions running smoothly, contributing to homeostasis. Not a lot is understood on how exactly the endocannabinoid system works, but it is known to be linked to metabolism, pain, inflammation, sleep, learning and memory, cardiovascular and reproductive system function, sleep and stress, as well as other functions. Whenever any of these functions are out of whack, the endocannabinoid system sends out its receptors, which are found in the central nervous system and peripheral nervous system, particularly in immune cells, to bring things back into alignment.

It is now believed that the euphoria felt during and after aerobic exercise, can be attributed to the activation of the endocannabinoid system initiating that "high" feeling post exercise, much like a "stoned" feeling post smoking marijuana, which is a version of cannabinoids found in cannabis. The release of endocannabinoids eases the mind and floods the body with feel-good hormones. It regulates other systems of the body making adjustments to bring anything that is needed back into equilibrium. Once the endocannabinoids have carried out their function and everything is back in balance, the body will then produce enzymes to break down the endocannabinoids to prevent any overcorrection.

The lymphatic system is part of the body's immune system and consists of a network of lymph vessels and lymph nodes. It is largely responsible in maintaining fluid balance and eliminating harmful substances and waste products from the body. The lymph nodes contain lymphocytes which attack and break down bacteria, viruses and damaged cells and deposit the debris back into the bloodstream to be further filtered through the kidneys or liver and disposed of through faeces and urine. As the lymphatic system doesn't have its own pump mechanism, it relies on movement to function. Smooth muscle tissue contracts to move lymph along through the vessels. Many lymph nodes are gathered near joints which assists the flow of lymph through the nodes by the means of a pumping action. As lymphatic flow is assisted by movement, it stands to reason that when we exercise, there is better clearance of pathogens and damaged cells supporting immune function and a more efficient mopping up of excess interstitial fluids maintaining fluid balance.

We live a more sedentary lifestyle than ever before. Our ancestors were always on the move building shelters, creating tools, hunting food and escaping from predators. Day to day living was mostly all about survival. People worked and roamed the land, swam and bathed in streams, rivers and coastlines. Constantly upright and active throughout the day, they would only sit to eat or work on their tools and lie down of an evening to rest, before a new day dawned and the activities of the day started over. As culture, society and technology expanded, man moved away from nature and had career choices other than farming, building and herbal medicine. No longer submerged in Mother Nature, inherent skills were lost. The great outdoors has now become a place reserved for leisure activities and relaxing and many jobs/careers, although not all, involve working indoors. Some of these occupations require little movement or activity. Interestingly, this movement of society away from nature prompted the introduction of forest bathing. More on that later. It is believed we no longer have the same unison of mind and body as our ancestors once did who were constantly swathed in nature.

Our sedentary culture involves long periods of sitting. Sitting at desks, computers, television screens, laptops and phone screens. Sitting in meetings, lectures, cinemas and restaurants. Most of us are just not moving around as much as we need, to support a healthy existence. When sitting, blood flow slows, diminishing oxygen supply to all of our organs including our brain, affecting our alertness, creativity, arousal, concentration and academic performance. Breaking up sitting time with even short bursts of movement can benefit health by activating our internal systems: blood flow, muscle contraction and insulin production. Prolonged sitting has detrimental effects to both physical and mental wellbeing. We need to keep on the move to benefit our cardiovascular function, our musculoskeletal and digestive systems and our flexibility and balance. Regular movement also promotes the production of feel-good hormones, increasing positivity and reducing stress.

It is easy to ignore our body signals when sitting for long periods, especially when transfixed by a screen, only to realise that when we do move, we find ourselves stiff and sore. We may be faintly aware of some aches and pains but they are readily dismissed when our mind is preoccupied, to acknowledge that we may need to correct our posture, or how much time has transpired. With busy time schedules and workloads to get through, even lunch breaks may be forfeited in favour of a quick bite at the desk. Switching from traditional desk chairs to stand up desks allows alternating between sitting and standing. Sitting on an exercise ball requires a constant balancing act which involves muscle activation and works on core strength. It is not necessary that you use these alternatives as a complete replacement for chair sitting but change it up a bit so that your body gets a semi work-out.

For someone with an office career, there is a lot of sitting down on the job. I used to hear that every cigarette smoked was a nail in the coffin and I have plenty of nails in mine after years of smoking. I have lived enough decades to reveal that smoking has most likely been a contributing factor to my medical conditions. Along with cigarette smoking, immobility is now equated to reducing life expectancy. Physical inactivity is known to increase the risk of chronic health problems such as cancer, cardiovascular disease, diabetes, musculoskeletal disorders, disease of the nervous and immune systems and neurological disorders. I can't erase smoking time. The damage is already done. I can thankfully choose regular movement over prolonged periods of inactivity. Yay!

A lifestyle that constitutes a predominantly sedentary time will still remain detrimental to health despite exercise. Exercising for an hour a day seven days a week won't iron out the risks associated with prolonged hours of sitting. Exercise needs to be constant and frequent. It is better to do small bouts of activity throughout the day than to wait until you get to the gym. A strenuous workout or an hour's walk or run, although very beneficial, won't undo the effects of prolonged physical inactivity. That's why it's important to disrupt sedentary time as often as possible by moving in some way: taking a walk or doing some stretches, bike pedalling at the desk or anything else that stimulates muscular activity. Periods of not being in motion add up subtracting from your health.

If you think of the daily life of an office worker, it may go something like this; commute to the office followed by an eight-hour desk sitting stint, then maybe a short walk to the car or public transport to commute back home. When home, there is some standing time while dinner is prepared, then it's usually back to a sitting position to chill out in front of the television screen before preparing for bed. And it all starts over the next morning when a new day begins. That day just racked up a whole lot of physical inactivity. But it doesn't have to.

Understandably, there may not be the time or inclination to undertake aerobic exercise of some kind but many moments of the day can be interspersed with some sort of movement.

Pelvic floor exercises can be done whenever sitting or standing. Stairs can be taken instead of the elevator. The walk from transport to office could be lengthened. Facial exercises can be done in the car. Just getting up from a sitting position to move around every 20 minutes or so counts. Our lifestyle is set around convenience. We have cars, remote controls and mobile phones and, as previously mentioned, many screens all of which favour stationary positions. We can get places faster on a set of wheels than on a set of legs and so, we often use automotive transport. Kids are often driven and picked up from school and there is more entertainment available for them that doesn't require movement. Chiropractors and physiotherapists are kept busy attending to muscular and skeletal problems that are more prevalent due to inactivity and poor posture.

Electrical activity in leg muscles shuts off as soon as you sit or lie down. Everything slows down. Calorie burning drops, electrical activity in muscles lessens and enzymes that help break down fat, diminish. Long term confinement to sitting or lying positions will eventually accelerate the ageing process as bone density reduces and muscle mass atrophies. Simply changing to a standing position massively increases energy levels and, of course, movement further increases these levels.

We have to be very mindful of how our sedentary lifestyle can impact our health and try to combat this by integrating as much movement as possible into our daily routines. Gentle activity, stretches, yoga, walking around and even fidgeting all contribute to increased delivery of oxygen to our cells and organs. Aerobic activity enhances this process, strengthening our respiratory and circulatory systems, as more oxygenated blood becomes available to carry out metabolic processes. If each of our body cells are powered with optimal oxygen the healthier our organs and systems will be, improving immune function and reducing the risk of cancer, high blood pressure, diabetes, heart and lung disease, stroke, obesity and mental illness.

Movement throughout the entire day every day is essential for sustainable health. It is not enough to make up sedentary time by periodically slotting in time for exercise. Aerobic exercise, whether it be moderate or of a high intensity, is fabulous for conditioning the cardiovascular system and, in effect, all bodily systems, which will help ward off disease, but it needs to be interspersed with frequent daily movement to gain optimal wellbeing.

One third of our lives is devoted to sleep where we leave the reality of our world and enter a land of slumber. There is a repetitive period of disconnect from our external environment in which we become unresponsive to stimuli retreating to our inner depths. But what is sleep really about and why do we need it?

Sleep is required to restore energy and regulate body functions. It is during sleep that the body gets to work on repair and rejuvenation, by cleaning out toxins, repairing tissues and replenishing hormones. There is a lot of work to be done during sleep to protect us from illness. In fact, the major restorative functions of the body occur at night during sleep.

The quality and quantity of sleep matters. There are several stages involved that repeat several cycles throughout the night. They include awake time, light sleep, deep sleep and REM (rapid eye movement) phases. Deep sleep is essential for tissue growth and repair, detoxification and strengthening of immune function and REM sleep is important in rejuvenation of the brain. Our bodies will transition between these stages according to our sleep needs. If particularly tired, we might skip the light phases and spend more time in deep and REM sleep. The body will work out the cycles accordingly.

During deep sleep, growth hormone is secreted by the pituitary gland which is vital for cell growth and repair. Our bodies are busy fighting off infection and inflammation during this stage of sleep. Certain antibodies and immune cells are produced as well as cytokines; a type of protein necessary in regulating immune function. The brain's glymphatic system, a waste clearance pathway, opens up and pumps cerebrospinal fluid (CSF) through its channels clearing the brain of toxic waste that has built up during the day. This process of elimination may contribute to a reduction in the risk of neurodegenerative diseases such as Alzheimer's and Parkinson's.

REM sleep is important for memory and learning and suppresses stress neurochemicals, making it easier to form memories and put them into perspective without the emotional attachment of the previous day's events. This may explain why, after a good night's sleep, the worry/anxiety you had the night before dissipates and you wake up feeling at peace, with clarification of a problem you may have wasted hours mulling over. Our mind downloads experiences of the day, files them, then awaits sleep to consolidate and sort them into memory and skill. Short term memory is converted into long term memory. Thoughts are sorted and stored according to their level of importance. The brain will erase anything that is not useful, to not clutter the nervous system. During sleep, brain activity is rife in areas that regulate emotion, which supports healthy brain function. We are all too well aware of how irritable, anxious and over reactive we can become when sleep deprived. Dreaming occurs during REM sleep where we are free from the confines of time and can create our own world, depending on where our thoughts take us in the vastness of our subconscious. We can do things in our dream life that are impossible in our waking life. We can fly, go back and forth in time and even visit with people who have died. We create our dreams where anything becomes possible. You are more inclined to dream more vividly or experience nightmares if you are sleep deprived, experiencing anxiety or on certain medications.

There are certain internal mechanisms at play that prepare the body for sleep and stimulants in our lives that can interfere with these processes. The two bodies that govern sleep are the circadian body clock and the homeostatic sleep drive. The circadian rhythm is a natural internal process that regulates the sleep-wake cycle. We have an internal biological clock that goes through a cycle every 24 hours. This is a natural cycle dependent on natural light and darkness. When the sun sets, melatonin secretion begins to ready our bodies for sleep. As the sun rises and we begin to become exposed to light, melatonin secretion stops and we become more alert as serotonin secretion takes over. Our sleep drive is our need to sleep. When we wake in the morning and are well rested, our sleep drive will be low but the accumulation of adenosine, a neurotransmitter chemical produced in the brain, over the course of the day will steadily increase our need to sleep. These two parties work independently to support our sleep regulation.

Circadian rhythms differ somewhat according to age but there can be disruptions that throw out the body clock, which can be difficult to reset. It is important to maintain as normal a cycle as possible, so the body gets enough restorative sleep to maintain good health. Melatonin is released during the night and suppressed during the day. Serotonin and cortisol are both responsible in stimulating wakefulness and supporting alertness throughout the day.

Body temperature drops and metabolism and breathing slow down during sleep as the body undergoes regeneration. It is important to create an environment that is conducive to these changes. Practice healthy habits. Avoid eating late at night and avoid stress and stimulants such as caffeine, alcohol and nicotine. Artificial light, including the blue light emitted from screens is a major disruption to melatonin production. Promote a comfortable sleep space that has good ventilation and isn't too warm. All of these things will enhance good quality sleep.

Modern life can upset circadian rhythms. Artificial light, technology, sleeping pills, travel, late night venues and night shifts can all disrupt the internal clock. Once dark, artificial light tricks the circadian clock and suppresses melatonin production affecting quality of sleep. A strong circadian rhythm will induce deep sleep and powerful cell regeneration, resulting in lots of energy. A blunted circadian rhythm will lead to poor sleep, incomplete cell regeneration and chronic fatigue and tiredness. Needless to say, the latter will cause undesirable consequences eventually increasing the risk of disease. The homeostatic mechanism or sleep drive, can override the circadian clock when there is a need for sleep. When sleep pressure is high, the body becomes less susceptible to light, which explains the ability to be able to sleep following a period of sleep deprivation, jetlag or nightshift. It is good to stick to or simulate as normal a circadian rhythm as possible. Apart from the illumination emitted from the moon, stars or campfire, all other artificial sources will upset our master biological clock.

Where possible, adopt regular sleep and wake times, refrain from using technology late at night and give the body time to slow down as nature intends it to. In the morning, open up the curtains or blinds to allow the sunlight to flood in, creating a normal shift in circadian rhythms bringing back a natural alertness as serotonin takes stage. Allow time to be in a full awake state before doing anything that places demand on alertness or attention.

There are obstacles that draw us out of sleep cycles affecting our overall quality of sleep. Snoring, sleep apnoea, noise, medication, bathroom visits and alarm clocks can all disrupt the amount of deep sleep we obtain, keeping us trapped in light sleep patterns. It doesn't matter how much sleep we tally up, if we can't move beyond light sleep, we simply won't get enough restorative sleep. Many of us rely on alarm clocks that can abruptly wake us from sleep. These can shock us into an awake state suddenly increasing our heart rate and blood pressure. Pulled from a state of calm to one of immediate alertness, there is no consideration of the stage of sleep we are hauled from. Natural light alarm clocks, otherwise known as dawn wake simulators, induce a more gradual wake up by using artificial light simulating dawn, thus keeping in tune with the body's innate rhythms.

Insomnia is a state in which our brains refuse to go offline, despite the best coaxing efforts from our tired bodies. We have all experienced this state of hyperarousal where it becomes difficult to align mind and body. Sometimes it's the mind that won't play fiddle and other times it's the body that refuses. Anxiety, fear and depression can raise cortisol levels which makes it difficult to get to sleep and stay asleep. Restless leg syndrome, pain, illness, insufficient exercise and poor sleeping habits can all contribute to insomnia. Apart from correction of any underlying issues, there are remedies to help calm the mind and help the body to relax to induce sleep. Things to try include a warm bath an hour before retiring, playing relaxing music or listening to mediative scripts, there are plenty available on YouTube and aromatherapy. These all promote endorphin release, calming the overexcited brain and have a natural analgesic effect on the body. If worry is keeping you awake, turn on the light and write down what you need to get done and pop it in the bedside drawer to stop you ruminating and wasting valuable sleep time.

Good quality sleep is critical to health. Wakefulness is a period when the body is constantly in alert mode, ready to make necessary adjustments according to environmental influences. Sleep is a time when stress is inactive, giving the body reprieve from being on guard. Cortisol levels naturally decrease when the body is at rest; paradoxically, high levels are counteractive to rest. It is important that the body is able to shut down and successfully doing so means toning down the sympathetic nervous system which is responsible for activating stress hormones. These stress hormones interfere with the production of serotonin and melatonin, necessary ingredients for relaxation and inducing sleep.

When we are fatigued, our brains can't function properly, affecting both our cognitive abilities and emotional states. We suffer from a decreased concentration span, reduced alertness, mood swings, problems with thinking and memory issues. Chronic sleep deprivation and poor-quality sleep can affect every body system causing cardiovascular disease, diabetes, high blood pressure and a weakened immunity. A weak immune function can lead to cancer, autoimmune issues and a host of other diseases caused by invading pathogens.

Good quality sleep requires conditions that allow the body to reach a level of comfortable slumber necessary for rejuvenation of all systems. Being happy and healthy correlates to creating such conditions and having consistent adequate sleep maintains the exact same state. Negative emotions, hyperstimulation, sleep disorders and illness can interrupt the natural sleep process and a lack of sleep can exacerbate these same conditions that are the root cause of insomnia.

The right diet, sufficient exercise and enough sleep are imperative to our health and longevity. Let's take a look at our chromosomal makeup to obtain a better understanding of how it all starts on a molecular level. There are little caps at the end of each strand of our DNA which protect our chromosomes called telomeres. These caps naturally get shorter as we age but they can also become prematurely shortened by poor lifestyle choices. Telomeres get shorter each time a cell copies itself and, over time, become too short to do their job, causing our cells to age and stop functioning properly. An unhealthy diet, sedentary life and sleep deprivation can produce oxidative stress and inflammation, accelerating telomere shortening, thereby increasing the risk of disease and reducing lifespan. Making healthy lifestyle choices has the propensity to lengthen our telomeres and longer telomeres are associated with fewer illnesses and a longer life.

It's ironic that the act of increasing productivity for a better lifestyle can in fact be a precursor for disease and a shorter lifespan. The aim to achieve, with the notion that it may make for an easier more remunerative existence later in life, usually involves making sacrifices. It may require working longer hours, opting for easy meal choices, skimping on exercise and reducing sleep time. There's no point in arriving at the end goal with a tattered body. The pressure to succeed can weigh heavily on health, insidiously reducing the number of years left to reap the benefits of all the hard work laid down, with the initial intention of creating a more prosperous life.

We can't be expected to be health conscious every day for the entirety of our lives. It's only human to slip up and indulge in unhealthy activities from time to time. That's okay. That's allowed. But for the majority of the time, if we improve our bodily functions through exercise and we top that up with a good diet and sufficient sleep we will be roaming the earth in healthy cloaks.

DEALING WITH STRESS

The human body undergoes stress on a daily basis. It is a normal physiological response to challenging circumstances. Stress is good for us. It exercises neurons in the brain improving memory, attention span and productivity. It also helps develop resilience. If we went through life void of any kind of stress, we would have no protective mechanism to shield us from dangerous situations that could threaten our existence. We are continuously challenged by changes in our environment and we constantly make adaptations to maintain a homeostatic state. Dealing with stress is a natural part of our existence and essential to our survival.

As in all animal species, man has an inbuilt automatic mechanism that protects him from any real or perceived danger, ensuring his own survival and that of future generations. When man was first assigned to earth, he spent a lot of his existence subject to the raw elements of his environment. He had to share his space with predators and didn't always have the shelter to protect himself against severe weather conditions. Life threatening scenarios were a part of his daily living and he had to constantly fend off danger. Luckily today, we don't face the same treacherous challenges but we do still work from the same survival instincts.

Our nervous system is geared to respond to threatening, challenging and dangerous situations. This enables us to deal with the prickly parts of life. To flee from situations that could cause bodily harm or endanger life and to increase alertness and energy required to deal with the peril faced. Some of life's thorns are bigger than others but they are never meant to be a constant hindrance.

There are two arms to our autonomic nervous system consisting of the sympathetic and parasympathetic drives. The sympathetic drive is activated when we undergo stress enforcing a state of alert and the parasympathetic drive brings us back to a state of calm. We have no conscious control over the workings of these two divisions. Each works independently, making necessary adjustments in keeping the body in a state of equilibrium. When there is a balance between the two drives, all body systems will run optimally.

When our sympathetic drive is activated, our flight/fight response kicks in and we redistribute fuel to our vital organs at the expense of shutting down other processes that are not required for defence. Stress hormones, called catecholamines and cortisol, are released which activate physical changes in the body to help respond to a stressful event. The airways of the lungs (bronchioles) open up, ravenous for more oxygen to deliver to the organs (heart, brain and muscles) which are conscripted to defend the body. Blood pressure increases as the heart pumps faster and stored sugars are loaded into the bloodstream. The body becomes equipped with fuel and strength to either tackle the situation or flee from it.

Once the stressful crisis is dealt with, the parasympathetic drive comes into play to revert the body back to a state of homeostasis, where all body functions return to normal. The parasympathetic nervous system is responsible for restoring the body to a composed state of rest and digest. Blood pressure eases and blood is redistributed to the organs that were compromised during the stressful event. Excess sugars are collected from the circulating blood to be put back into storage to conserve and restore energy. The body returns to performing its regular daily functions.

Our sympathetic and parasympathetic drives are equally vital to our health and survival but there must be a balance between the two for our bodily systems to function optimally. If stress isn't swiftly kicked to the curb, its hormones will linger, feeding a state of arousal which will, in effect, take a toll on the body.

Thankfully, we don't have the perils our ancient ancestors faced, but we have found plenty of stressors in today's world to trigger the exact same response intended for survival. You could say that stress responses are more often activated from a psychological perspective rather than from a life-threatening event. Sure, we feel something which activates a warning and our body automatically responds in the exact same way as if our life was in danger, even though it isn't. Much of what we become stressed over is only ever what we perceive to be a threat. More like a disruption to our lifestyle than a life/death situation. We can become all worked up over nothing much. And while we are fretting over these non-death causing scenarios, like trying to make a deadline and the mounting commitments we have on our plate, our bodies have lunged into a fight/flight state when it's not really necessary. Anxiety is enough to trigger the stressor hormones and the accompanying chain reaction that is designed for defence. And the more we become uptight, the longer the body remains in a state of alert. Sometimes stress is simply directed through our thought processes.

When our body reacts to a life-threatening situation, it can take 20-60 minutes for the body to normalise to its pre-arousal state. If you were to get a sudden fright you would immediately become aware of the associated physical symptoms: rapid heart rate and breathing, increased alertness and perhaps a feeling of being clammy and shaky. These are real symptoms that you feel and they settle down once the threat passes. What happens then if the stress is of a psychological nature? The telltale symptoms aren't always evident. You are more likely to feel anxious, moody, perhaps depressed and unmotivated, with an overactive mind of negative thoughts that you find difficult to hush. The fight/flight response has still taken place causing all the internal mayhem but without the on/off switch. Unless action is taken to reduce stress levels, the body cannot readily revert back to a pre-arousal state and so the stressor hormones are left to roam unabated eventually overwhelming the body and leading it toward disease.

It is inevitable that we will all encounter stress. It is how we manage it that is important. We will all react differently according to our particular temperament, past experiences and the resilience we have developed from previous incidents in our lives. Depending on our life experiences, we will all have varying degrees of response.

As you know, stress can be short term and long term, also known as acute or chronic. Acute episodes are short lived and the body returns to normality quickly. Acute stress is experienced on a daily basis. Being stuck in traffic or experiencing a near miss can heighten alertness and improve performance. Everyday pressures such as meeting deadlines, arguments with family, work commitments or a sudden illness, although short lived, may have a more lasting effect, especially if these stressors are repetitive or intense. Acute stress may turn into chronic stress when it is accumulative or extreme.

Unlike acute episodes of stress, chronic stress lingers causing the body to remain in high alert mode. Stress hormones swamp the body, increasing heart rate, blood pressure and muscular tension. The heart works harder as blood thickens, due to an increased production of red blood cells, cholesterol and high sugar levels. Cortisol, normally responsible for regulating metabolism and anti-inflammatory processes, is in overdrive causing multiple organ dysfunction and a suppressed immune function. If stress levels are abnormally high or persistent, then the body's ability to normalise is affected. Eventually the body can become overwhelmed if there is no regulation, as the stress switch is always on. The body can get so used to this chronic stress situation that it can go unnoticed. Feelings of agitation, hopelessness and low mood can become the new norm as the stress hormones insidiously take residence.

To protect our bodies from chronic stress we need to have an understanding of what our stress triggers are and how to manage our lives in such a way as to not burden our nervous system. In order for our body to run optimally, we need a balance between the two inputs. We don't want to sit in the emergency room of the sympathetic drive too often. As soon as we recognise that we are in it, we need to step into the healing room and put on our parasympathetic band-aids.

Stress is only ever supposed to be short term. It signals our body to adapt to challenges. Something occurs in our physical environment or within our thoughts to warn us of a potential threat to our wellbeing. This informs our body that we are subject to imminent danger and an immediate fight/flight response is activated. Within milliseconds, physical and biochemical changes take place. We are well equipped to deal with the disruption and once it is dealt with, we are meant to return our stress guns back into their holsters, to sit, ready for the next event. However, if these stress guns remain in our clutches, the body will continue to be in a state of alarm. They must be properly replaced to prevent accidental harm.

In today's fast-paced society where the stress response is constantly activated, it is increasingly difficult to return to a state of normality after a stressful event. Many of us still have guns in hand at the ready, anticipating that there will be another stressor just around the corner. Or worse still, have them fully loaded and constantly drawn.

Chronic stress is extremely disabling to the body, having serious consequences to our overall wellbeing. Ideally, we want our bodies to return to a state of equilibrium soon after a stressful event and to generally reduce our stress levels. To accomplish this, we need to identify our stress triggers and work on controlling them. Given the right tools we can handle stress before it takes a grip on our lives.

There's a lot to be done in this world of ours and we can be running around from dawn until dusk and even beyond, trying to fit it all in. Trying to keep up with daily demands and cram everything into one day can be impossible. It is important to prioritise ticking off the important things first, which may mean carrying over some other things on your list to another day or simply saying no to things that aren't essential. It is far too easy to become stressed by pretending to be superhuman. Take a break. Ask for help. An attempt to power through everything may cost you dearly. Not only will you be activating stress, you could be compounding its effects, as you will most likely be compromising on sleep, exercise and eating well.

Management and minimising stress are key toward optimal wellbeing. Reducing our daily demands and changing the way we think can reduce our stress levels considerably. It's not feasible to think you can get everything done in a specific timeframe. Your intentions may be good but as you know, unexpected events may crop up or you may simply underestimate the time you have available. Either way, there's only so much you can do. Accept that and give yourself permission to leave things for another time. Always give yourself some time out during the day devoted to relaxation, meditation or exercise. This is especially important when you feel stressed and panicked. Even though you may feel you can't possibly take time out of your busy schedule to indulge in yourself, the benefits are well worth it. Your sympathetic arm will try to dissuade you but just allow yourself to enter the healing room for a little while. Your parasympathetic arm will be there to greet you, soothing you of your troubles. You may find that after such a visit, your mind becomes clearer, solutions to your problems start flowing in and you start seeing things with a new perspective. You suddenly become more productive than you would have, if you hadn't taken a step out of your stress-filled day.

Our thoughts direct our body chemistry. Every thought produces a chemical reaction. We know that positive thoughts make us feel good and negative thoughts have the opposite effect. This is because our physiology changes according to the thoughts we think. When we think positive thoughts, we release serotonin, creating a feeling of wellbeing and when we think negative thoughts, we release cortisol, the stress hormone. Our perception of the world has much to do with the pathway of our thoughts. Sometimes we find ourselves caught up in automatic, negative thoughts (ANTs) where they can spiral out of control. These thoughts have a tendency to taint other random thoughts along their path, driving the momentum toward a negative mindset. Soon enough, stress hormones are activated and we feel tense and agitated. In a case of ANTs, thoughts have a tendency to grow more complex as they feed off one another. It is really difficult to switch off from this inner critical dialogue. On reflection, when we think back on our mode of thinking, we realise that our concerns were mostly exaggerated and in a different mindset, these concerns don't bother us anymore. Think about a time of having a serious case of ANTs interrupting you at night, cutting into your precious sleep time. Invariably, the next morning you feel cross with yourself for having wasted time on those kinds of thoughts when, with a fresh mind, it doesn't seem to matter at all. It's handy to remember that the actual process of sleep works on problem solving.

Besides setting up your body with stress hormones that interfere with your long-term health, negativity and negative self-talk will limit your ability to believe in yourself. It will affect your self-esteem, your potential and it will stunt your ability to succeed. You are more likely to be closed off to opportunities as your view of the world is clouded. Feelings of discouragement and depression may encourage unhealthy mind-altering behaviours. Optimistic, positive thinkers are less likely to slump on the couch and more likely to exercise, eat healthier and get more sleep than their counterparts. Their thought processes allow them to be less affected by stress and they are inclined to develop more resilience.

Thoughts direct our feelings, which set up our physiology which, in turn, governs our behaviour. Having an understanding that thoughts (which aren't often reality by the way) can shape the way we experience life, sheds perspective on how our decisions are often driven from within and not from the outside environment. To create change in our surroundings, we must first look within, paying close attention to our thought processes, as these determine how we choose to interact in the world.

Much of our behaviour comes from what's been programmed into the subconscious mind. In the first seven years of life, the subconscious mind downloads programs on how to behave. These programs come from the observations we make on how others react in the world and are automatically downloaded into our internal hard drive. Accordingly, we set up patterns of thinking which then become encoded in the brain. At this point, we have no control over our downloads. They may come from others playing negative programs, childhood trauma or stressors that we are raised on, in which case, we may have unconsciously downloaded dysfunctional programs which condition our automatic thoughts.

It can be difficult to rewrite our programs as our subconscious conditioning is always running in the background, telling us this isn't right, constantly reactivating our system and bringing us back to our old way of thinking. That which feels comfortable for us. Our wishes and desires come from the conscious mind, yet action often comes from subconscious programming. To update the software of our physiology, we have to engage the conscious mind in an effort to change any negative conditioning and rewire our system to improve the quality of our thoughts and hence the quality of our lives.

The subconscious mind holds all our conditioning,

positive and negative. Sometimes we may become aware of what lies beneath our surface when something in our outside surrounds conjures up a thought or memory. This will have an emotional attachment. We can't relive our past but we can acknowledge that the software created from it, may compound a stressful situation. We are capable of redirecting our thoughts to create positive behaviours and positive outcomes.

Focus your attention on your thoughts and be aware of how they affect your mood. Catch yourself when engaging in negative thinking, notice any tension or stress that thought process causes and change your thought pattern. It can be difficult to just stop, so allow yourself a limited time to wind up those thoughts and then switch to something more positive. If you are mulling over a concern, maybe it would help to imagine yourself as if you were simply an onlooker, which may help you detach from the associated emotion and give you more clarity. Think of how you will feel in two days or one year from now. Will it matter then? Is what you are thinking grossly exaggerated at present? Try reframing your thoughts with a positive approach.

To keep stress at bay, it is important to keep tabs on our thoughts which have an enormous influence on our body chemistry. Your thoughts don't necessarily reflect reality but they will cause real changes in your biology. The body will react to whatever the mind perceives as being real and this can come from a thought, suggestion or emotion. Notice how sometimes you become aware of the tension in your body when you are watching a horror or thriller movie. Of course, you know it is just fiction but that doesn't stop the reaction you are having. Just as automatic as a loud noise causes a startling effect. Your body has reacted before your mind has differentiated between what's real and what isn't. Recognise how your body reacts and then make a change to create a flow of feel-good hormones. I'm not saying don't ever watch those types of movies but if you have a lot of stress going on, you could change your biochemistry by switching to a comedy or nature documentary.

Approach life's challenges with a positive outlook. Positive thinking sets up a positive physiology and we want to nurture this. Choose to focus on positive thoughts and pluck away at any negative conditioning which is not only limiting but can cause disharmony that can eventually lead to disease. Make a change to a positive frame of mind, so you are predominantly residing in your healing room.

We can avoid unnecessary stress by being instrumental in our environment. Some things will happen to us that we have no control over but we can select our reaction to these events. There are other things we can be selective of. Set yourself some boundaries and know your limitations. Surround yourself with positive relationships: people you can confide in and talk things over with, people who make you feel loved and upbeat. Limit associations with people who are negative or demanding. These people don't often give you a fair exchange; they monopolise your time and siphon your energy. Their aura can be toxic to your own emotions. Afterward, you can come away feeling drained and that feeling can stay with you for a far longer period than the time spent engaged with them. Understand that it is their own mindset coming from a place of dissatisfaction and protect your own by maintaining your emotional distance and limit your expectations of them.

Know when something is unchangeable. There's no use feeling frustrated after devoting too much time and effort to people who give you little in return. As it's not always possible to eradicate unhealthy relationships, neutralise their toxic effects by spending less time with these people and use your armour of positivity to protect your inner peace. You have your own share of stress to deal with. No need to load your plate with anyone else's.

We all need a time of rest, a time in which we can put aside things that require our attention. We will always have some things on our "to do list" so there is no use trying to power through, thinking we can get it all done in a nominated time. To free up some space, you may need to adjust your standards or enlist some help so you can concentrate on the important things. Taking a break can help slow down your pace and prevent you from becoming overwhelmed. It is better to step aside from tasks, demands or commitments, as that way you will remain on an even keel rather than giving the stress hormones free run, causing havoc throughout your body.

God created a sabbath day for rest because on it, God rested from all the work he had done. He created a commandment: Remember to keep holy the sabbath day. A day of worship intended for rest and restoration and reflection on uniting with God in our eternal resting place – heaven. Why, you might ask, would God, who is almighty and powerful, need to rest? He didn't. But he included rest in the law of his 10 commandments, knowing that's what his people would need.

Despite individual religious beliefs, Sunday used to be a day where we could shut off from the world. Non-essential services were closed. So was the case when I was growing up. There was nothing much to do and I remember it as a day of quality time spent with family as everyone was home. There were no computers or personal devices to retreat to. After a leisurely lunch, we'd take a Sunday drive or play a game of monopoly that would run well into the afternoon. Otherwise, we would laze about doing nothing much, hoping that the Sunday night Disney movie would be a good one. It was a guilt free day of relaxation and it felt great. Now Sundays are pretty much like any other day of the week and, with so much to get done, it's difficult to allow ourselves a complete day off, so it is important to make a conscious effort to set aside at least one sabbath day of our choosing to rest and recuperate.

Creating a day that is totally void of commitments, a day with which you can do whatever you please, is respite for the mind. After such a break, you may find that you have become more resourceful, coupled with a renewed enthusiasm when you take back your responsibilities. If you think you can't possibly afford a day off, think again. Take a look from an outsider's perspective. If you were your own best friend, what advice would you give yourself if you noticed that this person, you, had become overwhelmed with life's daily demands?

Life is a constant challenge. We all have hurdles to leap over at times. Stressors in life certainly create discomfort and uncertainty but there is always something to be gained. Instead of worrying over life's difficulties, consider them tests designed to help you grow and expand. It is only by forging ahead that we cope through adversity and learn resilience, through which we develop an inner strength. We carry on. We get better at jumping the hurdles. If we avoid tackling our difficulties, we won't rise above our problems. New concerns will join the party causing overwhelm and we may find ourselves on an escape route down Mind Numbing Lane, indulging in unhealthy behaviours that temporarily soothe our incessant negative mind chatter. These ANTs, however, have the ability to rise above their shackles and stomp on any logical thoughts, leading to chronic worry. Issues become a lot more difficult to deal with as the management toolbox becomes depleted and we may plummet downward into a state of anxiety and depression.

If you find that stress is getting the better of you, it is important to seek out some strategies to help you manage it. Meditation is a practice undertaken to still the mind and it is something you can practice on your own. Just take some time out of your day to focus on quietening the mind. This involves giving yourself permission to let go of all that needs to be done and realigning with your inner being. Start by focusing on your breathing, allowing random thoughts to drift in and out of your mind. Sit quietly. As your mind relaxes, you will discover a heightened sense of awareness. Notice the temperature of the air and the stillness of the objects around you. You may notice the blueness of the sky and the gentle rustling of the trees as you gaze out the window. Tune into your senses, dismissing any thoughts as they try to barge in. Think of how you feel when you are in a place of nature.

Nature in its peace and beauty can ground us. We may feel our anxieties and concerns dissolve in the wonder of its vastness and the true connection we have with it. As humans, nature is what we first identified with and it's amazing how relaxed we become when we are removed from the world of cement and steel and of all else that is manufactured, mechanical or electronic. In fact, forest bathing originated in Japan in the 1980s as a means to relieve stress by connecting to the healing power of nature. The psychological and physiological benefits of spending time in nature have long been recognised to improve mental and physical health. What better way to wash away the trials and tribulations of life than to immerse in the natural world? Time spent at the beach, a picnic in the park or camping/hiking in the wilderness is not only enjoyable but a restorative, meditative experience. If you think you don't have time for engaging in such activities/experiences, think again. You'll be detoxing your mind and body and revitalising immune function, all of which accounts for wellness and longevity.

Yoga, similar to meditation, is another way of reducing stress. It involves a connection of mind, body and spirit, unifying the body as one in harmony and giving us a true sense of balance and oneness. Yoga comes in many forms, incorporating varying poses and exercise. There are classes you can take in person or you could just find a suitable one on YouTube. Other ways of de-stressing include engaging in exercise, laughter and humour, massage therapy, music therapy, hypnotherapy and aromatherapy. You may have also heard of Emotional Freedom Technique (EFT), also known as tapping therapy. It involves tapping on specific acupressure points of the body; invisible pathways to unlock emotional blocks and restore energy balance. It is used for both physical pain and emotional distress. The stimulation of meridian points through tapping can release associated stress and negative emotions, freeing the body of tension.

Endorphins are your feel-good natural opiates that are released in abundance when you partake in any of the above-mentioned activities and therapies but you can also activate these wonder hormones by adjusting your thinking process. Thoughts translate to an associated emotion so you can reconfigure any thoughts that cause trepidation. Engage in positive thinking and let go of bitterness, anger, envy and guilt. Practice gratitude instead. Your body will instantly become doused in positive hormones. Remember that your mind will become blocked in a negative state and flourish in a positive state.

Don't be overcome with worries. As you know, you can employ counselling services to help you manage stress. Sometimes it's enough to share your feelings or talk something over with a trusted relative or friend, so that stress doesn't become overwhelming. Understand the underlying causes for your feelings. Adjust your standards. Forgive yourself and others. Make it a priority to service your body physically, mentally and spiritually. Remember to take regular breaks of uninterrupted time-out for yourself, spent on relaxation and self-indulgence. When we obtain an inner peace, our nervous system becomes more balanced, opening a wide spectrum of opportunities that enhance our capabilities and lead to feelings of contentment and peace.

HAPPINESS

What is happiness and where does it come from? Happiness is defined as an emotional state characterised by feelings of joy, satisfaction, contentment and fulfilment. I think you'd agree that we all strive for happiness in our lives as it makes for an easier, more pleasurable way of living. But how do we get there? What can we do to acquire joy in our lives and sustain contentment? Is this desired state of being something we acquire through things we possess, through experiences we encounter or is it something that comes from an inner satisfaction deep within?

One thing for certain is that happiness is obtainable at any time, regardless of our circumstances, gender or status in life. There exists a misconception among some, that happiness is only achievable at certain times such as when a person marries, purchases property, obtains more wealth, accumulates more possessions, loses weight, takes a vacation etc. We well know the feeling of elation when any of these things occur but it is only ever transient. At some point, we adapt to our new circumstances, return to baseline and go in search of something else that boosts our level of happiness. In an attempt to stimulate our pleasure centres, to obtain that "high" we may get caught in the chase rather than settling for contentment in the moment, as we seesaw between highs and lows. These ongoing pursuits do contribute to happiness, however, there is a more enduring form that creates long lasting inner fulfilment.

Health is an important factor in happiness. If we are suffering in some way, physically or mentally, it is more difficult to achieve the same level of satisfaction we may otherwise have in a state of complete wellness. We can choose to eat healthy, sleep well and exercise to favourably contribute to our wellbeing. Eating the right foods, being physically active and getting enough sleep flushes the body of toxins, improves immunity and is an open invitation for endorphin release (remember they're those feel-good hormones that counteract stress and boost mood). If we are in good health but miserable, the negative emotion of misery will reset the body's biochemistry offsetting all of the stressor hormones, which when persistent can lead to a multitude of conditions and disease. If you are doing all the right things keeping physically fit, then it's diddly-squat if your mind is on another planet. Body and mind need to be in alignment to maintain a state of wellness and wellness is a main ingredient of happiness.

There are people in this world who are terminally ill, yet happy. How can this be? You may wonder. We sometimes see stories in the news or in social media of individuals who have been given the "death sentence", smiling and enthusiastically detailing things they are going to do on their bucket list. They seem so calm in the face of adversity, it seems incredulous. Studies have revealed, these people are more connected to gratitude. They see every day as a blessing and are more in tune with their inner being, as time ahead is unknown but definitely limited. I'm sure their focus is entirely on what they can receive and give out to the world and so they maximise each and every day.

Sometimes illness is unavoidable, despite all our best efforts in trying to maintain health, and some of us have to live with chronic disease. Maintaining a happy disposition, having a positive attitude and focusing on good nutrition, adequate sleep and exercise, as well as seeking support and having a good knowledge of the illness, will all help in sidestepping worry and getting back to some normality of living that constitutes deriving satisfaction and joy.

How do we find enduring happiness, moving from short-term gratification into long-term gratification? A sense of inner fulfilment is attained through gratitude, acceptance, a defined purpose, well-developed compassion and forgiveness, of ourselves and others, and altruism. If our thoughts direct the way we live, we should focus on abundance in life rather than scarcity. Our ability to enjoy life comes from how we think and how we view ourselves in the world.

Spirituality enables us to move away from the perception of just being a physical body in the vastness of existence, to a connectedness to something much bigger than ourselves. It is a belief that we are a part of a greater whole, cosmic or divine, that defines our entity. It could be described as a sense of oneness of consciousness that abides in peace and harmony with all things. Spirituality is our central core and it has no beginning and no end. Here we reside in a deeper realm, which allows us to find purpose and meaning in life and to be in touch with our intuition. Spirituality involves a deep sense of interconnectedness to the power within us, the universe, God, a higher power, whatever you believe it to be. Spirituality deepens our sense of prosperity in life. It goes beyond money to include the appreciation of health, love, relationships and time.

Cultivating spirituality entails experiencing quiet reflections, connections to the moment, to nature and oneself. It can involve private prayer, meditation and yoga. When life is viewed as more than just human sensory experiences, there is more meaning attached and a trust that the higher power has us covered. This gives us a sense of security and we are less likely to worry, be angry, bitter or jealous or focus on ourselves, which equates to being generally happier.

It is easier to exercise gratitude if we are able to view the world from a bigger perspective, rather than from a place of our own wants and needs. That way, we are open and receptive to abundance, switching off from the notion that happiness can only occur from a succession of pleasant episodes or material gains. Practising gratitude puts the brakes on seeking more. It accentuates that life is precarious, that nothing is promised and all that we have in the moment needs to be treasured. Place your attention on what is happening around you right at this moment and aim to appreciate, respect and value it, as much as you believe is possible. If you find it difficult to be grateful for what you have right now, think of how it would be if something was taken away from you. I'm sure you have experienced that sense of panic and disappointment when you have misplaced or lost something of value to you, followed by the delight in its return? You have a renewed appreciation for something you took for granted. Make a habit of consciously counting your blessings. Gratitude has the power to block out negative emotions and encourage positive thinking and behaviour, which leads to an optimistic outlook and a greater satisfaction in life.

I have experienced gratitude in a way I wouldn't have thought possible. In the passing of a loved one. When a dear friend of mine died from a sudden illness, close people in his life, some of whom I knew well and others whom I had just met planning his memorial service, formed a meeting group to commemorate his life. Periodically, we gather together in a social setting, often at the venue on the beach where we had his service and floated candle-lit lanterns out into the sea. Sometimes, he comes with us in a canister but, otherwise, I consider a little piece of him residing within each one of us and it feels evident at each event. Even in death, the beauty of the person remains and the appreciation of life is celebrated, heightened by the soul that simultaneously passed but remains always present, anchored in our hearts. We come together, grateful for all that this person contributed to us in our lives, sharing the connection and love.

People strive to obtain material goods in order to feel better about themselves, believing that once acquiring a fill of possessions, they can sit back and be satisfied. Yet nothing is owned or lasts forever and time is consumed in looking after material possessions. Time is valuable and, if some of it is lost in this way, then there is less time available for human relations. We can easily get stuck in making comparisons. A competition begins, hell-bent on acquiring something better than a friend, neighbour, family member or whoever else. It is as if the worth of a human being can be measured by the acquisition of things. In an effort to feel valued, you must continue to replenish your supply of material items. This leads to an endless pursuit for more. It becomes difficult to keep up and eventually the endless pursuit for more becomes too much or too competitive, which conjures dissatisfaction, rather than satisfaction. Ceaselessly comparing what you have against what others are accumulating is futile, as there will always be someone with more than you and someone with less.

To be able to experience any form of happiness, we need to keep check on our emotions. It is normal and healthy to experience all emotions positive and negative but our minds tend to amplify the negative. To prevent an avalanche of negative thoughts flooding the mind, take some time to deal with anger, guilt, envy and sadness or whatever negative emotion you are experiencing. Deal with your feelings, release them before they have a chance to burrow deep within where they may fester causing resentment, bitterness and depression. Take anger for instance. It's something we all experience from time to time and it can and should be released, in a healthy way. If someone was the cause of your anger, confront them. Confronting the person who caused the feeling provides empowerment over the emotion. Despite the outcome following this consultation, forgiveness will realise the emotion further. Don't hold on to grudges, allowing resentment to take residence. You have the right to acknowledge pain and regret. Do so and then allow it release. As difficult as it may be, if you don't allow negative feelings release then you are in danger of becoming shackled to them. Life can only move forward and those feelings are now past, so let them go. Screaming at the top of your lungs, preferably in your own space or punching into the bed or pillows are great ways of releasing anger. Just get it out. Instead of letting thoughts ramble in your head where they distort and gather power, write them down and rationalise a response. Once on paper, you can look at them objectively and unravel the distortion they caused.

There are behaviours, our own or others, that we resent.

We cannot go back and change anything in the past. We only have control of now. Forgiveness includes acknowledging the pain and regret these unsavoury behaviours may have caused and then releasing them. In the case of your own, let them go; you have the power of change. In the case of someone else's, also let them go; you have the power to change how you feel. Allow yourself to let go of any resentment by forgiving yourself your mistakes and the hurt that others have inflicted upon you. It is the only way to find your way back to peace and harmony, allowing happiness a chance of survival.

As mentioned, some stress is good for us and in small amounts it can build on our resilience which can overall increase our potential for happiness. Take, for instance, the process of working toward a new goal, changing careers or learning a new skill. These situations can definitely cause stress in the interim but once victory is reached, personal gain is evident and this sense of accomplishment ignites happiness. Having to deal with moderate stressful situations in our lives sharpens our focus and activates an immune response. Once the stress is over, we feel more confident and ready to take on another challenge. This can boost our productivity and build our resilience with similar future incidents. From time to time, we will experience brief periods of stress in our lives that cause concern about our health or livelihood. These too, can be categorised as having a positive outcome, as it is when we come back from a traumatic event that an ordinary day seems a lot rosier. We are relieved that that event is over and we get on with our lives with an added spring in our step.

Chronic stress is ongoing and accumulative and can't easily be shaken. This form of stress not only causes havoc on the body leading to disease; it can also be responsible for dis-ease.

A feeling of uneasiness or distress occurs which barricades any form of happiness. It is vital to deal with stress as it happens, so it doesn't have a chance to overwhelm the body. It's not always easy to switch off from chronic stress, especially if you become so accustomed to it that you don't even realise you are switched on. Activities that should relieve stress and create a sliver of sunshine in a dull day, can, in fact, be too difficult to undertake in a depressed state of mind. There is a lack of energy and motivation to even contemplate partaking in the usual stress soothing remedies.

Perhaps it would help to list the causes of stress in your life at this present time. You may be surprised with what you come up with. If they are broken down into bite size pieces, you can start to tackle them one by one. Remember to talk things over with trusted family or friends or a healthcare professional, who will help you gain perspective and enable you the emotional support and motivation to take action. Whenever you can, allow some joy into your day. Take a stroll through nature, eat chocolate, take a relaxing bath, watch a comedy – anything that will enhance your mood, just enough to bring your body back to a state of calm. If you practice doing something every day, no matter how small, you can start to chip away at your stress and begin to return to a healthy state. When you make a start, you will find your motivation trickles back in and you can then upsize to more enduring stress relieving activities. Don't forget to get plenty of sleep, eat well and incorporate some exercise into your day.

I believe much of our happiness is under our personal control. Optimism can help enormously in dealing with life stressors. Life's difficulties are easier handled if we hold onto faith that there is also a silver lining. All things in life are transient. There will be good times and bad. Overcoming challenges requires being selective in your thought processes. If our thoughts drive our behaviour then it makes sense we will have a better footing during life's hardships with a positive attitude.

We are all vulnerable to suffering. It is a part of life that carries no immunity card. We will all experience loss of loved ones, illness and ageing. We can learn to cope by drawing on our resilience, accepting that life is ever-changing and that deep within, we have the strength to bounce back. People enter and depart from our lives leaving behind valuable lessons, gifts of love and memories to carry us forward. Illness can enhance our spirituality and, as we age, we gather a repertoire of wisdom. Having an appreciation of these personal gains allows us to rise above our pain of loss and permanent change.

It is the way in which we view things in our world that will determine our reaction to them. It is pretty easy to be deluded by the unfortunate circumstances of life with a pessimistic mindset. There is a propensity to highlight negative events, assume the worst and be suspicious of anything good on the horizon. Pessimists are more inclined to think that life happens around them and they don't have control. They are less likely to reach out to others for help and risk becoming insulated from life to protect themselves against anything worse happening. Their fear of the unknown is too great to enter uncharted waters and so their dreams and aspirations may lie dormant. Many doors remain closed in the house of the pessimist and their ongoing negativity takes a toll on their mental health, which of course will spill over into their physical wellbeing.

Optimists tend to fare better in life than pessimists simply because their attitudes differ. They have a positive outlook on life exercising control over events. Difficulties are regarded as temporary and there is a focus on other aspects of life that denote gratitude, keeping everything in perspective. Positive thinkers don't retreat into a shell when things are difficult, instead they approach problems as opportunities and remain socially connected, seeking help if they need it. They are more inclined to step outside their comfort zone to tackle challenges and, in doing so, they build on their creativity and resilience. Optimists are popular, they are easy to be around and this attraction promotes happiness and stability. Many doors open in the house of the optimist and new doors are created. Their positive mind-set promotes physical and mental wellbeing with a tendency of a longer lifespan than their counterparts.

Happiness may feel unobtainable when we are suffering stress, loss or illness. Our upbringing and experiences in life can predispose our thought processes. In a negative mindset, difficult situations can lead us to believe our lives are limited, undermining our self-worth and crushing our potential. When we change the direction of our thoughts to a more positive outlook, we see things differently and the walls of our restricted vision begin to expand. Creativity is accessed and, 'I can't do,' becomes, 'I can,' as we tap into our resources. One of the most powerful ways we can develop resilience and enhance happiness is by thinking optimistically.

As humans we are a social species. We thrive on social interaction and require intimacy with one another to promote a positive sense of wellbeing. To enhance our relationships with others, we firstly need to be comfortable with our own being. The way we relate to ourselves ultimately determines the way we relate to others and the way others relate to us. Our relationship with ourselves sets the tone for every other relationship we have. Rather than seeking perfection and carrying a mentality of not being good enough, we can be accepting of who we are and work toward achieving goals of self-improvement. Self-acceptance is essential in achieving inner fulfilment through which we can develop meaningful relationships with ourselves and others.

Happiness involves loving and accepting yourself unconditionally, which includes being content with your life as is, without yearning to be someone else or have someone else's life. We all have our individual life journeys equipped with our own set of gifts and quests that make our lives unique. Instead of carrying regret or wishing your life to be different, make use of your special qualities and talents. When you take a close look at the hand you have been dealt, you will discover that you have the power to embrace your life circumstances by drawing on your inner strengths. Infinite opportunities are available in life if we are accepting of them; they carry us forward, providing insight and wisdom. Life can be unfair at times; it's the nature of the game. Remember, it's not singling you out; it's the way it is for everyone. Make the best of what you have in hand and don't let limitations define your existence. It is only when we surrender to the ebb and flow of life that we can obtain tranquillity and contentment.

Experiencing true happiness is significantly enhanced when we feel connected to and enjoy the company of others. These connections can be transient or long-term. When we are involved in healthy relationships, we sense a feeling of belonging, of being appreciated, accepted and loved. We have people to support us and with whom we can confide. We are more inclined to build positive relationships when we have the right relationship with ourselves. We can't totally rely on others for our happiness; that needs to come from within. Others can, however, add enormously to our sense of joy and fulfilment.

A higher level of happiness can be achieved by carrying out good deeds and genuinely caring for others. Have you ever felt a lift or deep sense of satisfaction when you display acts of kindness, generosity or compassion? These acts activate all those feel-good hormones: endorphins, dopamine and oxytocin, keeping us in parasympathetic mode; a state of calm which will ultimately steer us toward optimal wellbeing. Oxytocin is known as the bonding/love hormone enhancing our connections with others. Altruistic deeds can strengthen our relationships and are known to boost our mood, so if you are feeling low, the act of helping someone might just give you the lift you need.

In order to achieve long term gratification, it is important to set some goals in life. It is so easy to just allow life to happen, putting a few plans in place along the way. Setting goals allows us to focus on our desires and dreams and gives us the motivation to work toward these. Pursuing life goals requires a concentrated effort of hard work and is bound to conjure up feelings of fear, self-doubt and anxiety, which is why we often retreat to the procrastination bench. But the longer we stay seated, the less likely we are to grasp hold of opportunities and our dreams will just become fabricated notions never manifesting into reality.

When we have set goals, we have something to work toward and an end result to look forward to. Not all our goals may come to fruition but constantly having something in place provides organised structure and establishes our sense of purpose. Exercising our creativity and utilising our resources gives us a sense of achievement and satisfaction, which can lead to greater success and performance. Once we embark on accomplishing our goals, we gain confidence and find more opportunity cards come into play. Along the way, we connect with new goals and through those that resonate with us, we may define our life purpose.

A sense of purpose adds meaning to our life. It means being able to live life to the fullest. Purpose is crafted from our personal values and desires and ignites our passion. It is an ongoing pursuit that gives us reason to get out of bed each day with enthusiasm, as the challenges and tasks we undertake arouse our authenticity and contribute to the betterment of our world. Having meaning in our lives sustains us, even during times of stress or when life becomes tedious. When we are working toward our personal goals, investing in our interests and unique talents, we have something to fall back on when life takes that unexpected turn. Something that keeps us motivated can reduce the impact of chaos in our lives.

Your purpose in life is as unique to you as mine is to me. We may share similarities to others, however, what becomes important to you that gives your life meaning, is designed from your own personal attributes. It could involve a major project or a series of smaller projects. It doesn't have to bring you fame or fortune or change the course of the world. It just needs to be worthwhile and meaningful to you. To be able to recognise your gifts and employ your abilities creates a tremendous sense of satisfaction and can also strengthen human connections. If your inclination is to hold back on something through fear of failure or what others might think, listen to your voice within. Trust in your intuition, it will lead the way. It is your inner light that taps into your ultimate wisdom.

When we are in connection with a project or activity that

captivates our interest, we can enter a state of flow, where we are so immersed in what we are doing, we are oblivious to everything else. We are totally connected to the moment, completely absorbed, mind chatter silenced, as we completely unite with the activity. In this state, there are no hindrances to distract us from extracting pure enjoyment from our activity. Self-awareness slips away and time has no meaning, when we are totally involved in something we enjoy or have a passion for. Having a purpose in life can create flow-states which is the epitome of living in the moment. When we are challenged and involved in projects that have meaning for us, we are generally content. We have purpose in our lives.

Living in the moment allows us to extract the very essence of life. So often, we are caught up in mind chatter pulling us away from the present. We mull over regrets from the past or worries of the future. We can become so accustomed to these intrusive thoughts they become difficult to silence and we find our bodies immersed in the present and our minds – somewhere else. There was a time before our mind became so preoccupied with thoughts, that we were fully immersed in the moment. Remember being a child when all that belonged to you was now? How good did that feel? You utilised all your senses and in doing so, extracted all you could from the present. When I recall being a child, I can remember soaking in everything. My mind had space; there weren't any relentless thoughts distracting my presence. I hold vivid memories as my senses intensified my experiences. Today as an adult, I often have to apply a concerted effort to stay in the moment.

It's difficult to just stop thinking but we can train ourselves to be more present in the moment by practising mindfulness. It's really just about being planted in the "now". Thoughts come and go; we can't completely silence the mind but we can reduce our thought processes by tuning into our senses. When we acknowledge our thoughts in a non-judgemental way, we don't let them sabotage our ability to connect to the present and we can once more delight in all that we feel, hear, smell, taste and see. Unencumbered by cascading thoughts, we are free to experience the curiosity and astonishment we had as children. Life then becomes unveiled as our connectedness to everything in it strengthens. The more present we are, the more enriched our lives will be and the better equipped we are to form memories to take into our future.

Moods differ every day according to life circumstances. We can't be expected to be in a good mood all the time. Sometimes moods are unpredictable. A sudden unexpected outburst may reveal that we are on edge, resulting from a bad night's sleep or, having been so busy, we have had little down time for ourselves. There are many mood enhancing therapies, some of which are better for us than others. Healthy coping habits work on naturally changing the brain chemistry to promote the flow of feel-good hormones. Meditation, yoga, talking things over, exercise, spending time with your special people and many other things can lighten your mood. One of the most enjoyable stress relievers is to partake in an alcoholic beverage, as long as we don't get too comfortable in drowning our sorrows away. It is very easy to self-soothe with mind altering activities or substances, however, it is best to do so in moderation as it can induce an artificial change in brain chemistry that can skew normal circuits.

Self-medicating or self-soothing with illicit drugs, alcohol and nicotine mess with the normal intricately orchestrated, neurotransmitter circuits of the brain. Normal neural circuits are disrupted as these substances latch on to neuron receptors augmenting the release of numerous neurotransmitters in abnormal amounts. This creates a heightened neurotransmitter response and an accompanied false sense of pleasure and reward is experienced, due to an overstimulation of serotonin and dopamine, the neurotransmitters affecting mood. These intense euphoric feelings initially experienced, motivate people to repeat the same behaviours and, in some cases, an addiction may result. Over time, if these substances are continually used, the brain becomes accustomed to the changes in brain chemistry and there is an overall decrease in normal dopamine and serotonin production. This has an effect in lessening the satisfaction from once-pleasurable activities. The resulting physiological changes in the brain can lead to an impulse to continue to consume substances to reinstate the normal reward circuits. To complicate matters further, withdrawal of the substance to regain normality can backfire by activating stress neurotransmitters. Just another trigger to entice one back to the very substances that cause a fake reward, just to regain some sort of equilibrium. A vicious cycle begins.

Tampering with the neurotransmitters by the above-mentioned substances can potentially have a long-term impact on our mood and general health affecting our happiness. Other self-soothing, mind-numbing activities that could become addictive and detrimental to health and happiness include: excessive eating, gambling and shopping. Although these activities feel good at the time, the consequences of weight gain, debt regret and feelings of guilt and shame, certainly don't.

Once a person steps on the merry-go-round of addictive behaviour it can take some serious modification to correct, which often involves therapy. It's not just a matter of taking a look at oneself and thinking, 'I know this is bad for me, people are judging me and I need to change, this is embarrassing; I am a fatso, alcoholic or druggie – I look terrible, I have no money, my friends and family have abandoned me.'

Addiction is an illness that surpasses the point of self-indulgence and plummets into a loss of all self-control. The dependency becomes so overwhelming that sickness, loss of self-respect and status, simply aren't enough to hoist one out of the abyss of hopelessness.

Attempting to change the physiological chemistry of the brain through natural means is far more favourable than with medication. Some people are believed to have disruptions in their neurological pathways and require medication to simulate normal functioning of their neurotransmitters. However, these people and their medications need to be monitored carefully as there is no accurate method for measuring chemical levels in the brain. There is no known evidence that anxiety and depression are caused by a chemical deficiency, but administering medication that increase levels of serotonin, dopamine and norepinephrine (neurotransmitters) have been found to alleviate symptoms. Biological, psychological and environmental factors may all play a part in mental illness. It may be a combination of things but it is not correct to say that it is chemically related, nor is it known to be entirely incorrect. There are too many chemical reactions occurring in the brain all at once, that it is impossible to pinpoint a singular chemical imbalance. Unfortunately, there is no control over the collective function of the neurotransmitter targeted with prescribed medication, so there are unwanted side effects. For those people with transient or mild forms of anxiety or depression, alternate therapies may be considered as the preferred first line of treatment. Hypnotherapy, psychotherapy, yoga and meditation can work on channelling thought processes which can effectively work on modulating behaviour that favourably alters brain chemistry.

Life can get testy and, at times, it just becomes too much to bear on our own without some kind of assistance. Sometimes our pride gets in the way of asking for help and so we go about pushing through, trying to figure it out for ourselves. We are grown-ups, we don't want to appear needy or out of control or admit to our failings. Perhaps our failure to reach out has to do with the very loss of perception that our circumstances have caused. It is undoubtedly difficult to rise above the insecurity and doubt we may feel without putting aside our egos to let help in. We are all here for each other and sometimes we just need to reach out for a hand to allow healing to take place and stroll back along the path to happiness.

There will be times in life when we have to put happiness on hold while we deal with significant losses: death, divorce, separation and illness. These may also include: loss of a job/career, financial stability or losing a dream or goal. As we work through our anguish and grief, we learn resilience and draw on our inner resources. These difficulties can elicit all that we have to be grateful for, shedding light on things we may have previously taken for granted. It is sometimes through sorrow that we fully appreciate the joys of life.

There will always be episodes in life that will increase or decrease our level of happiness. It is impossible to feel 100 percent happy 100 percent of the time. And that's a good thing as, if we were always perched up high on our pedestal of happiness, what would we have to look forward to? What would we strive for? It is when we work through challenges and solve problems that we feel a sense of achievement. And, yes, achievement and success often involve pain, devotion and sacrifice but that is what drives our purpose. We can't hang around doing nothing, expecting change or that everything should remain the same. We need to roll the dice and play the game.

We are continually learning and gaining insight from our personal life experiences. If your reality is different from what was desired, so be it. Accept that your life path is indelibly yours, that requires drawing on your own special strengths. Turn mistakes, regret and pain into valuable lessons rather than let them eat away at your integrity. They are there to give us the opportunity to look deep within ourselves and change aspects of our being. This soul searching can lead to a fuller, more satisfying, life. When we discover our inner potential, we may revalue the cards we have been dealt.

True happiness needs to come from within a person, not from the outside world. Enjoying life in its entirety involves living in the moment and, to achieve this, we need to peel back the layers of our conditioning before our ego distorts our perceptions, as it is only then that we can experience an inner joy untainted by self-judgement. There within, lies abundance from which emerges deep fulfilment.

PART FIVE

• • • •

Surprise Cards

LIFE HAPPENS

Wow, look at that! These hailstones are the size of golf balls! OMG look at all those cars parked in the street, including mine. I hope they aren't damaged. These were my thoughts as a loud pounding sound summoned me to take a look outside. Hailstorms of this magnitude are rare and my astonishment temporarily overrode any thoughts of possible destruction this pelting from the sky may cause. Once the storm ceased, I tentatively went to inspect the aftermath. Under the twilight grey of the sky, my car appeared undamaged. Or so it seemed. I reinspected it the next day. Whoa! The hail had hammered the car. I resigned to paying the $800 excess it would cost me on my insurance claim, my inner mind cursing, 'Damn, this wasn't my fault! This bloody act of nature is going to cost me money!'

Alas, the car was deemed a total loss. Now magnify the cursing. This was the first brand new car I had ever purchased only three years earlier. All my previous car purchases had been second hand models. I wasn't ready to update and didn't want to replace it with a second-hand model. What to do?

Eighteen thousand dollars was the estimated quote given for fixing the car. Well really, it's cosmetic features. Seriously, I could get a facelift or multiple plastic surgeries for that. Stuff the car's exterior, I would rather improve mine. I would much rather spend my hard-earned cash on my own appearance than on the appearance of a metallic possession. Who really cares how a car looks? It was no worse than a bad case of acne scarring. My choices were: to keep the car or claim the insurance and buy another. The first option was perfectly reasonable as, mechanically, the car was sound. However, the dilemma would be to accept that it had lost all value, making it difficult to resell and near impossible to regain comprehensive insurance. On these grounds, I chose to purchase a new car. Sixteen thousand cars were damaged in that storm, on that particular day in the district in which I lived, many of which were deemed total losses.

It has always baffled me why society values the appearance of a car. We are quick to fix any imperfections from minor scratches to major dents. Does it really matter? Unless the damage affects the performance of the vehicle, it's really just a blemish on its surface. Yet, we are between a rock and a hard place as any damage sustained equates to money lost when it comes to reselling the vehicle. That's the way it is, so we ride with it and either pay the money to fix the car or suck it up and continue to use our car, accepting its imperfections along with its loss of value and possible effect on insurance coverage. Somewhere along the way, we have perhaps become too obsessed with the appearance of our automobiles. Most of us sport some scars on our bodies that can't be perfectly rectified, so we just live with it, however, when our car sustains imperfections, we are quick to seek a reputable panel beater to cosmetically fix its features.

Life happens and acts of nature can interrupt life's course, causing a temporary derailment. Unexpected events of any kind or magnitude will cause a diversion and demand adaptation to new circumstances. Life constantly sends us challenges, testing our integrity, faith and humanity.

Stones, rocks and boulders are thrown in front of life's path and we duck, run and sometimes get clobbered. Pebbles, although more easily dodged, can trip us up, interrupting our course. These pebbles can be classified as nuisance mishaps: wine spilt on the carpet, a ball thrown through a window or a flat tyre. Annoying as they are, they are temporary diversions. Boulders, on the other hand, can obscure the way ahead or create a tortuous route, requiring life to hit pause mode in order to deal with the impact these obstacles cause.

Picture this; you wake up in the morning in a fine mood and start to think about your day ahead. It's pretty straightforward – breakfast, work, home, dinner, relax, bed, sleep, or maybe the day is entirely free for you to do with whatever you wish. You may expect little diversions throughout the day such as having to attend an appointment or meeting, call in on someone, refuel the car, pick up some supplies or whatever else. But you don't usually anticipate the common mishaps that may throw you off keel: the sauce splash over your shirt, the public transport strike or the sick child. These "what ifs" aren't consciously factored into your day. They are unexpected mishaps, causing setbacks in your planned schedule. Even though they are small bumps in the road, it's a hassle to slow down or veer around them, particularly if your day is already tightly packed and you can't afford the time these misadventures demand. Let's say, these are the pebbles and stones of life.

On any given ordinary day, you may be subject to a much bigger setback in life: the loss of a job, a major illness, death of someone close, an unexpected pregnancy or any major incident or accident. These types of events can cause you to feel temporarily disassociated with life. A protective numbness may envelop you, protecting you from other distractions, as you figure out a way through the disruption. We'll call these the rocks and boulders of life.

Sometimes everything happens at once. You may be busy weaving your way through the boulders that have obstructed your path only to discover stones being hurled at you. What the hell?! You figure you already have enough to deal with without any other dilemmas thrown in. Is this God's joke? Huh, this could only happen to me, right? It may seem that you have been singled out for bad luck. In actual fact, everyday mishaps will occur spontaneously, at any given moment, to you, to anyone, despite what you may already be dealing with.

When you already have a full plate of hardships, any add on mishaps may be more difficult and frustrating to deal with, which intensifies the effect they have on you. Something as simple as peeling the shell off a hard-boiled egg can be enough for you to lose the plot when you don't get the membrane. Not normally warranting a justifiable outburst but, in your current state of mind, it can be enough to carry you over the edge.

Life goes on regardless of when it rains, pours or hails on you. It doesn't wait for you to run back for your umbrella. You have to deal with its unpredictability and make adaptations. There is no point in dwelling on the unfairness of it all; it's just the way it is. Chaos happens in life. It has nothing to do with whether you deserve it or not. It happens anyway.

DEALING WITH WHAT LIFE SERVES UP

Life is unknown and can suddenly take us all by surprise. All at the same time. We cruise along, expecting we have freedom of choice but that can be abruptly taken away from us when the world has a crisis to deal with. Our ancestors have lived through major disruptions with world wars, lethal diseases and famine. We can become complacent when we have lived in a world that hasn't had a global crisis for decades until suddenly it does. We are well aware that people in our past have had to live through and deal with extreme events, such as dividing loved ones and revoking freedoms during war or disease, but it seems incomprehensible in today's world. Now, even with advanced technology and scientific knowledge, we are faced with major viral diseases to combat, which affect the way we go about our daily lives. Just in recent times we were all sitting ducks under the pandemic umbrella of Covid-19.

Personal setbacks are challenging enough but something on a global level takes on a new dimension as it is out of our personal control. Heads of government, advised by the World Health Organisation (WHO), made decisions for us by which we had to comply in an attempt to minimise the spread of infection. A viral disease that originated in China caused chaos as the rest of the world looked on and, as it swept through continents, authorities tried frantically to put measures in place to halt its spread. Controlling the disease rode on the speed and effectiveness of decisions made by individual countries. Still, the virus moved in mysterious ways and sometimes faster than measures could contain, putting our health care systems under enormous strain. Not only was the virus demanding more intensive care beds, it was bumping those patients who equally required those beds for unrelated serious illnesses. People were forced to go into lockdown, to stay at home to presumably stay safe. This stepping out of normal societal function has had a crippling effect on worldwide economies and has subsequently led to an increase in physical and mental health issues. This you all know as you have already seen the pandemic unfold.

It is incredulous to imagine that something invisible to the eye can cause such worldwide devastation. Microscopic terrorists playing such havoc on the world. A virus can cleverly hijack a human cell and decode it with its own genetic material conforming the cell into its own replicate. Once its genome is released into the host cell, the virus then targets neighbouring cells and the process is repeated. This minuscule microorganism rapidly clones itself to form an army within the body, insidiously destroying all healthy cells in its path. To stop this genetic recoding and eventual massive destruction, the body calls upon its defences and a war begins.

The body is equipped to deal with many parasites, bacteria and viruses that cause illness by deployment of the immune system. Every illness causes an immune response which, in effect, strengthens the body's protection against future pathogens. When the body is exposed to a germ, the immune system will carefully examine, memorise and code a response to it, so the next time the same or similar germ enters the body it has the infrastructure to go into combat and destroy the invader. In other words, it builds an immunity. The immune system has constant exposure to many pathogens and with each infection it encounters, it builds a resistance to protect the body from future cell destroying diseases. The more practised the body is in building immunity, the better equipped we are in fighting future disease-causing pathogens.

A highly contagious disease, Covid-19 started in one person and that one entity inadvertently transmitted the disease to others and it soon became a world pandemic. When a virus is new to the human species, as this one was, there is no pre-assembled defence as the body has no recognition of the pathogen, no built-in immunity or antibodies to neutralise the virus and so it goes into full combat to eradicate the virus. The body also needs to analyse the virus to form a resistance or immune response to the offending organism. Immunity prevails the majority of the time, however, there are cases in which the body can't adequately defend itself and the virus wins the battle. The body doesn't know what to do with the virus and, in an attempt to devise an appropriate defence, the immune system pulls out all measures and is sometimes sent into overdrive creating an exaggerated response or cytokine storm, which may further complicate the effects of the disease.

As the cellular terrorists are left to multiply unabated, our only defence has been to keep out of their way, keep our distance from their far-reaching tentacles by isolating from others and optimising our battle fields by building a strong immunity.

The intense focus on the novel coronavirus created worldwide apprehension and mayhem. Never before had governing powers all around the globe put together such rigid rules regarding the way we live. Our freedom and liberties were quashed. We had rules to follow. Consequences were put in place for non-compliance. This change in lifestyle caused suppression of economies, distrust toward governing powers, as well as blame and control. Lockdowns inadvertently caused social isolation, loss of businesses, bankruptcy, an increase in mental illness and domestic violence and delayed diagnoses and treatment of serious illnesses. Being cooped up indoors may have even worsened the severity of the illness as the immune system is weakened by an insufficient amount of vitamin D, derived mainly from exposure to sunshine. Not to mention the associated stress causing a rise in cortisol levels suppressing immune function.

Theories have surfaced pertaining to the origins of the virus. Was it manipulated in a laboratory? Many questions have originated regarding the lethality of the virus. Reflecting back, did the collateral harm of the disease managed exceed the threat of disease and death related to lockdown? Was it really as deadly as predicted? Were the statistics correct? Were there flaws in the testing system? Do masks and distancing really work? And what of the vaccine being rolled out before the completion of clinical trials?

Covid-19 altered the way people lived their daily lives. It took away many liberties. It affected us all. No matter what theory you or I or anyone else has, we had to live through what life served up. The human race has survived many contagious diseases leading to important breakthroughs, scientific discoveries, the development of vaccinations and the improvement of sanitation and hygiene. In the 14th century, the Black Death signalled the idea of quarantine: the discovery where isolating people prevented the spread of disease. Cholera led to improved water sanitation and in 1980 WHO declared a worldwide eradication of smallpox by a collaborative vaccination program. All of these pandemics had high mortality rates.

Look at history, what we have already endured and have come through. In a time when the world was less sophisticated and underdeveloped, compared to what is now. Our world has advanced and we still have pandemics to combat. This won't change and I am sure this will go on for decades and centuries to follow. It is all a learning curve necessary for advancement in technology. There are tremendous gains from new discoveries and humanity continues to benefit from these.

Thankfully along the way, health experts have learned and are still learning more about the disease and have developed therapeutic treatments which have proven successful in lessening the severity of the virus. Vaccines can assist the development of immunity to an invasive pathogen and we are now well into the stages of administering novel vaccine technologies for Covid-19. Scientists are continuing to study the virus and its evolving variants to fine tune treatment.

So, here we are, living in times in which we have had to make some radical changes to our normal routines. We were inundated with news broadcasts on all matters pertaining to this pandemic and it was pretty easy to get fed up with the disruption to our daily lives. As frustrating as it was, there are positives to be gained in all of this.

Whenever something skews our life path, we have to change tack. Take on a different direction. We have all experienced this, as each of us has already had personal quandaries, setbacks and hardships. When life presents a challenge larger than one on a personal scale, all we need to do is apply our coping mechanisms that it has previously taught us. We need to distinguish between what we can and can't control and make the best of the situation we're in. There are always uncertainties of the future. This has always been and always will be, so there's no point in stressing over them.

Having the world shut down is like closing the curtains between stage acts. It can give us more of an interval to reflect and be grateful for all those things that have caused complacency in our lives. Sometimes it takes something being taken away from us to appreciate what we had. Priorities change. There comes a shift of what is important to us. As we step off the treadmill of life and give ourselves some reprieve, we become acutely aware of the simple things in life, from which we derive pleasure and satisfaction. Experiencing periods of lockdown or isolation can free up some time to take on a project or get things done that we have left on the back burner for far too long. It can bring out our creative side. During Covid-19 walking became one of our only forms of outside activity, and gyms were replaced with online versions. Perhaps now it has encouraged exercise otherwise not undertaken, had we not had the experience of lockdown. Going without during isolation can renew the appreciation of human contact giving relationships a chance of rekindling when the world reopened. We live in an advanced world where we can keep in touch in many ways through digital communication. No doubt we have all become a little more computer savvy than we once were and, since the video conferencing app Zoom expanded during

Covid-19, learning and meetings can now still be elected to be conducted from home.

Lockdown or isolation demonstrates how important it is to keep our minds busy and maintain human connections. I am not underestimating how difficult being in isolation can be, as it can and we all have our own challenges. All we can control is our perspective on how to deal with it. Usually, we whinge about not having enough hours in the day and we have now come back full circle to that and, now the tables have turned, wouldn't we just like a little more free time Covid-19 afforded us? Some of us may have felt frustrated with too many people in isolation together or being in isolation alone. Hopefully this pandemic has taught us to factor in more downtime in our lives and to prioritise our relationships.

During Covid-19 restrictions most of us were in and out of lockdown, quarantine or isolation to have felt the relief and pleasure of being rewarded by the activities that we had otherwise taken for granted. Restrictions barricaded our normal recreational pastimes. Our toy box was intermittently placed under lock and key. All of the things we once took for granted now have a heightened appreciation and exhilaration attached to them as they had been taken away and then given back. Being able to once again socialise face-to-face and attend public places: cinemas, pools, sports games, gyms, restaurants and playgrounds, allows us to reflect on all that we have to be grateful for but in the whirlwind of life didn't previously stop to realise or fully appreciate.

Perhaps there is a big life lesson in all of this. This pandemic forced us to slow down, rethink our priorities, enjoy and participate in activities that, if not for lockdown, we may have otherwise forgone. It has perhaps given us a deeper understanding of the hardships the lonely, homeless and elderly face. Hopefully, there exists a change in humanity for the better.

ILLNESS

Illness is one of life's humps. Unpredictable and sometimes unavoidable. Most of us will suffer illness to some degree in our lifetime. It could be acute or chronic and range from a minor to major health event. The best line of defence to prevent or manage illness is to choose a healthy lifestyle. That way, we can prime our immune system to do its ultimate best in dealing with disease causing illness and chronic conditions. Diet, exercise, adequate sleep and reducing stress and toxin consumption all contribute to the way in which we shape our body's defence system. The more shields we erect, the more protected we will be against invaders disturbing the mechanisms that keep mind and body in a tranquil state of equilibrium.

Avoiding as many environmental assaults as possible can strengthen immune function. You've heard it all before: avoid smoking, minimise alcohol consumption, avoid getting fat, eat well, sanitise to avoid picking up infection causing bugs and, when applicable, vaccinate against virulent pathogens. There is much we can do to get our immune army marching, incorporating all troops and this is good, very good, however, unless we live in a sterile bubble, we will always be subject to environmental elements and toxins, slowly chipping away at our defences. Recognition of this is imperative in selecting good habits over bad and taking precautions where possible.

Coping with a serious illness can pull the rug out from under your feet. It can crop up unexpectedly and leave you with a host of emotions to deal with, when all you want is to pretend it never happened and get back to the life you were living. Just a moment ago. Before you became aware of this disturbing upheaval. How could things change so dramatically in a split second? If only you could climb out of the human cloak that has suddenly weighed you down with a ton of lead and slip back into the non-diseased previously issued version, so you can carry on as normal, once more feeling comfortable in the skin you're in. Denial, anxiety, isolation and a blatant reminder of mortality, is enough to feel frozen in your tracks and, somewhat or completely, detached from the world as you process this predicament life put you in.

I was admitted to hospital recently to undergo a second round of neurosurgery – vascular coiling. The first part of the process involved an angiogram to get a detailed look at my multiple cerebral aneurysms. On admission, I was more anxious than I anticipated. As a nurse, I am usually the one rolling the blood pressure cuff around the arm, simultaneously gathering relevant information and delivering explanations. Not that person about to don the white gown and plastic wristband. I was passed the all-too-familiar gown and informed of which way to wear it. Whenever I have been a patient, I have always notified the staff of my profession. Not to be a smarty pants. No. Just so they know I have an understanding of "some" things, to make their job a little easier, without the associated cumbersome explanations on things mutually understood. Nerves distorted my cognition. I put the gown on back-to-front. Idiot. I hadn't felt particularly nervous about this preluding procedure up until this moment. It was the next one in line that I was concerned about. Was my anxiety premature or was it that I felt out of control being on the other side of the fence in this role reversal situation? Guess I'm just as human as anyone else.

Blood pressure high and pulse racing, I felt somewhat embarrassed and annoyed with myself that self-meditation just wasn't working. I know these techniques well. I teach self-hypnosis skills to pregnant women when I take them through the hypnobirthing program, for god's sake. So why couldn't I calm my own nerves? I needed to pull my nervous system out of sympathetic drive and park it in parasympathetic mode. This, I know you can do by simply changing a mindset. Nope, my mind wouldn't budge, no matter how I coaxed it.

When you are in sympathetic drive, you are pouring out stress hormones and, while these flood your system, your thoughts formulate the worst-case scenarios. Everything is accentuated. It's like your senses have erected a million hypersensitive antennas. Honed in on everything. Paranoia sets in as you hold on to every word spoken and try to decipher what is meant by 'that tone of voice' or 'that silence' or the extended view given to your medical notes or images displayed on screens. All the while, your eyes desperately try to perform gymnastics in order to steal a glimpse of what it is that's so concerning. Wait, what's that forward leaning gesture to get a better view? Yikes! What the hell is wrong? Things become distorted as negativity dominates your entire reality. The mind behaves illogically and you can't stop it. The illusion you create is totally convincing.

Any illness underlines our mortality. We can't assume that

perfect health will accompany us throughout life. There will be times of sickness. Not only in ourselves but in those around us. People we hold dear. Family members. Other loved ones. We have to face it upfront. Nurse our own illness by listening to our bodies and taking the time to really care for ourselves, resisting the urge to push through. Support and nurse those whom we love through their illness, without jeopardising our own emotional and physical needs. As a carer, it can be extremely draining and when every ounce of strength and courage is spent, it is easy to fall into the pit hole of exhaustion, so it is vital to take breaks. Where possible, give yourself some respite, take some time out for exercise and leisure and make sure you get plenty of sleep. You may need the support from family and friends to be able to refuel. You're not superhuman so accept all offers and, if they are not forthcoming, ask. It may be helpful to join a local carer support service and link into any relevant support group chat line.

When I was diagnosed with cerebrovascular disease and a heart block, I chose to modify my way of living. This wasn't easy and it took time to make changes. Habits that are life forming can be difficult to break. I had a go at it. I gave up smoking but would still have the occasional puff. As smoking went hand in hand with drinking, it wasn't as difficult to minimise my usual alcohol intake. Which, I might add, was a regular indulgence. I initially didn't make any real changes to my diet as I thought that cutting out these two vices was a mean feat. Along the way, as I was clocking up on years, I decided that I had better cut out the cigarettes completely and look at a healthier diet and lifestyle. So, I did. I partake in an alcoholic beverage very occasionally. I make sure that I don't skimp on sleep. I had treatment for my sleep apnoea.

I exercise regularly and, where possible, I try to avoid stress causing situations and thought processes. Yes, I have made changes but I can't say that I always strictly adhere to them. When living with chronic health issues, it was easier to pretend that they weren't really an issue, especially when there weren't any associated symptoms. Thank God our outer appearance changes as you age, a true indication that life has an expiration date and was enough to prompt me into action.

There are illnesses that some of us have to endure over a lifetime. Chronic conditions that may not have a "cure". Diabetes, hypertension, cystic fibrosis and lupus to name a few. These conditions can, however, be monitored on a day-to-day basis and managed by acquiring a good understanding of the condition through education, adopting a healthier lifestyle, along with support from health care practitioners and linking up with people who have similar health issues. Let go of self-sabotage. If only I had lived my life better, taken more care, not been so reckless or whatever else. There is no use for blame. Only change. Change in habits. Change in attitude. It is easy to adopt healthy envy, when you watch others indulge in what you cannot. Thankfully, a change in lifestyle generally means you are working toward a more fit, more productive you. You may find this change benefits other aspects of your overall wellbeing. The dividends are well worth it, from feeling better, to living longer.

There can be a wide range of emotions to manage in the event of a chronic or serious illness. Work out what helps you deal with these emotions in a positive way. Focus on taking the time out for yourself to do this. Latch on to those who are prepared to help and support you and let go of those who are of little benefit to you. It is sometimes through illness or some other serious life event, that the true essence of relationships is revealed. Time is precious and energy can be low and not everyone, including family members, may understand or be supportive of the challenges you face. Some relationships can just add stress to an already stressful situation.

As a caregiver to a loved one with an illness, it is only normal to have challenges and difficulties that are inherent in close relationships. These can be magnified with the stress that comes with caregiving. Tiredness, irritability, worry, and tension can be wearing and exasperation can spill over into outbursts, followed by tremendous guilt for having lashed out at someone so seriously ill. Take breaks. Share the load, if possible. Talk it over. The sick won't want to feel as if they have burdened you. Explain and apologise. Fortunately, love is unconditional and we are inclined to take liberties with those closest to us. Although this is generally understood, the seriously ill have surrendered their independence and can feel guilty for the physical, emotional and financial pressure they are exerting on their family/carers. Understand that they are in a vulnerable predicament. Where possible, give them back their independence. Families, although in all goodwill, are unaware of how suffocating they may be on their loved one, when they take on more than is necessary.

Illness may require the use of strong pain medication which include prescription opioids. Opioids are a derivative from the word opium, a product of the poppy plant from which pain medications originated. Opioids have the propensity to be abused leading to addiction, causing fear among the ill and their carers. Of course, health care practitioners are careful when prescribing medications to patients who have a past history of addiction but if you have an illness that requires strong pain medication, the chances of becoming addicted to prescribed opioids are exceedingly low.

On her diagnosis of mantle cell lymphoma, I asked my mother's doctor for a prescription of sleeping tablets to ease her anxiety and allow her to obtain some beneficial sleep. On picking up the prescription of temazepam (yes, a habit-forming medication) I was surprised to discover that the packet of blistered tablets was cut in half. Ten of the usual pack of 25 tablets were administered. I was furious. My mother had to deal with a newly diagnosed life-threatening illness and was only given a miniscule amount of medication to help relieve her nerves. The fear of a patient developing an addiction, which is highly unlikely, especially in the case of no previous alcohol or drug abuse, overrode a holistic approach to patient care. What added to my fury was that Mum waited 90 minutes over her appointment time to receive a diagnosis.

Already fearful of the prognosis of a large lump in her axilla, the GP emptied out her waiting room leaving mum until last. I can assure you that this supercharged our anxiety levels. The "dis-ease" caused by anxiety can create havoc on an already compromised state of wellbeing. Delivering the news of a serious illness can be awkward, especially when the prognosis is grim or unknown but being kind and honest and reassuring the ill person that they will be well looked after, can offer tremendous relief and support. Words, attitudes and behaviours, can have a profound effect on how critical information is received which, in turn, can determine the impact the disease has on the quality of future living. It is important to treat the person as a whole, focusing, not only on his or her physical needs, but emotional and spiritual as well. Being diagnosed with a serious or chronic illness can paralyse a person's ability to think rationally as they come to terms with their condition. Thrown off kilter, they may surrender their independence to others and lose confidence, trust and faith, as they search for a way back to some normalcy. With no other choice than to succumb to the confines of their illness, autonomy can be lost along with identity. There may be a period of withdrawal and depression. All this needs to be acknowledged and respectful care can reinstate dignity.

All people, despite their incapacities, have the right to be treated with the same dignity that they once had before they became ill. Some sick people have accompanied dementia, are old and frail or intellectually or physically disabled and it may be assumed they are not in their "right mind" to be perturbed by any changes or even grasp what is happening. That is no excuse to be lax on privacy or dismissive in any way.

If you or a loved one are diagnosed with a chronic or life-threatening illness, learn all that you can about it. And I don't mean through searching on the internet. You need trustworthy sources. Seek out information from health care practitioners, join support groups with others in the same boat and discover ways of improving your own health so you can support your body in coping with the disease. The more empowered you are, the more confident you will be and this will set a positive body biochemistry. Your thoughts and beliefs are capable of producing chemicals required for healing. It is important to keep the body in a calm, harmonious state, employing the parasympathetic nervous system, which is necessary for rest and repair. Taking control of your health, following your intuition, releasing suppressed emotions, embracing social support and deepening your spiritual connections, can all have a tremendous impact on healing.

Drop all negative thoughts as they will flood the body with

toxic chemicals deactivating the immune system. When you are anxious or stressed you upstage your sympathetic nervous system. Adrenaline and cortisol are activated as the fight/flight response takes over. Blood is redirected to your vital organs as in a primal sense, your body prepares to fight back or run away from a dangerous situation. The heart needs to pump faster, increasing blood pressure and pulse rate and your brain needs added fuel to sort out a plan of action, often overthinking, causing distress. The body is in alert mode ready for action and, while this is the case, there is less blood perfusion in all other organs of the body and processes that aren't immediately essential are suppressed. The immune system shuts down, digestion slows and toxins are left to clog up in the body, having no process of elimination.

Focus on healing, which may not guarantee elimination of your disease but will help you live the best life you have. Your body may be beyond healing but your mind and spirit may still be intact. Remember that mind, body and spirit are all connected, so you can work with what you have, to create a state of peace and balance. Engaging in meditation, prayer and a host of natural therapies may not bring about a cure, but rather an acceptance of the illness and help ease physical and emotional pain. As shocking, depressing and scary a diagnosis of serious or chronic illness may be, life is to be lived. Undo the shackles holding life back and grasp onto the raft that can keep you afloat through all the challenges ahead.

AMBIGUOUS LOSS

In this life we will all experience loss. Some losses will be recognised by others and some won't. Ambiguous loss can be of a very personal nature and not always evident to others. These losses can sometimes be undermined as they don't always have a clear definition, nor are they scaled in any way in order of significance.

Ambiguous loss can be unsupported and misunderstood. Unlike the loss of a loved one through death, there is no such ritual, like a funeral, to validate the loss, so it may dangle for a while until the sufferer acquires the means of dealing with it. The nature of the loss and how it is perceived by others, if it is indeed recognised at all, will determine what support structures, if any, are offered by professionals, the community or family and friends.

A divorce, an illness or a missing person tend to gain empathy from others as they are in the category of substantial losses. A child moving on, a falling out or separation from a spouse/partner, family member, friend or a partnership, or a relocation to another state or country, can equally cause substantial grief, however, as these losses aren't as tangible as others, the individual can be left to suffer alone in silence.

There are many losses throughout life that are real to us

but unrecognised by others and so we tend to deal with them alone, often believing that because they are unrecognised, they don't warrant the attention of anyone else. People can be misguided assuming that death is the worst kind of loss. However, loss through divorce, disease or a family estrangement or disappearance, can be just as devastating. Even though the loved one may still be living, they are lost in every other sense. This loss is somehow considered less devastating than death when actually it should be considered on a parallel.

The significance of loss can only be categorised by the person experiencing it. Some people move from one state or country to another for varying reasons and the loss they experience for what they leave behind will differ for each of them. In the case of fleeing a war-torn country, an abusive relationship, a life full of despair or a lonely existence, the emotional consequences may be mixed – grief may be wrapped in an anticipated hope for something better. If the relocation means a career opportunity or transfer or stepping out to experience another world but leaving behind familiarity, a loving family and a group of close-knit friends, then the move can feel bittersweet.

Substantial grief can be experienced as a result of missing out on something expected in life, such as: failing to achieve set goals, never falling in love, never marrying, inability to find a lifelong partner, disintegration of a proposed lifelong relationship, inability to have children, including pregnancies that have terminated, failed IVF attempts and stillbirths, having a disabled child or inability to add another child to the family. The list goes on. The desire for something never gained can be all consuming and unnoticed by others. This ambiguous loss is probably the most silent and others, oblivious to the inner turmoil experienced, may inadvertently make a comment that rubs salt into the wound. When a loss is recognised, such as death, disfigurement or loss of a bodily function, then tongues are held out of respect. No one would announce their marathon achievement in front of a paraplegic bound to a wheelchair. However, unbeknown to others, someone might be silently grieving loss of a personal nature and are vulnerable in a world where others unassumingly take things for granted. They are unarmoured, without means of protecting themselves against the emotional trauma they are carrying. It may seem that everyone else gets to dance in the Garden of Eden, partaking in the fruit that is cruelly forbidden to them and it hardly seems fair. To add insult to injury, others oblivious to their sorrow, don't make any attempt to conceal their delight as they prance around enjoying all that the garden has to offer.

Maybe life changes dramatically following an incident which impairs an ability once taken for granted. The loss of sight, hearing, communication, comprehension or ambulation, can greatly impact normalcy once known. A period of grieving accompanies adjustments to a new way of life. These losses may undoubtedly cause other losses in life: job, relationships and independence, so mourning for something once had can be a double whammy.

Unfulfilled dreams and hopes can cause a period of unexpected grieving. It is not uncommon for parents of an only child to pour all their hopes and dreams into the future of that child. As with any parent they want their children to succeed in life and when there is only one child to focus on, these expectations may become paramount. Perhaps they have unfulfilled desires of their own that they were unable to accomplish and so they hope to achieve their dreams through their offspring, as that would definitely be second best. Despite all the support, encouragement, education and money spent on the child to prime them for their expected pathway, disappointment may ensue if that child takes on a different path than what was desired or what the child was groomed for.

Ambiguous loss may be experienced by absentee or busy parents. Children are very reliant on their caregivers, usually a parent to love, approve, guide, support and nurture them in their developing years. They require the presence of a parent or significant other in their lives on a daily basis. The amount of sufficient time a parent spends with the child on this basis will be determined by the age and requirements of the child. An older child won't require constant attention that a young child demands, however, it is as equally important to be available. If a parent is constantly absent from their child's life, either physically or emotionally, then the child is bound to suffer in some way. This loss can be particularly detrimental to the child's emotional wellbeing. Even though the child will feel the loss, immaturity can make it difficult to comprehend the emotional consequences and, hence, when the child is grown, there still remains a small, fragile child that occupies the body of an adult with unresolved issues and an underdeveloped maturity to make much sense of it all. This emotional immaturity and neglect can interfere with normal healthy development, narrowing the window of life opportunities. In the body of a child, this type of loss is incomprehensible. And when the child is grown, immaturity may stifle reflection, preventing such a loss to be fully realised.

Absentee parents will also experience loss. Circumstances may interfere with time spent or the ability to bond with their children. Work or social commitments, exhaustion, dealing with emotional trauma or stress, inability to display affection or being too busy in their own activities including headspace, can all lead to an inability to form a healthy relationship with a child or simply enjoy their being. Time travels quickly as childhood takes a sudden turn into early adulthood and, as a parent reflects, there are bound to be regrets: moments missed, being too harsh or too lean, being preoccupied or inattentive and, most of all, the amount of quality time spent with them. It is only on reflection that we truly see how precious children are and how limited childhood is. A parent's hope is that they have provided enough for their children to evolve into healthy, successful and balanced human beings and to create many memorable snapshots to treasure, well after their children have left the nest. The ultimate aim is to form a bond that is strong enough to weather all storms, creating a profound connectedness that remains forever present, even in absence.

Absentee parents risk missing their children's milestones and growing years. The chapters in a child's life are short and there is no replay. Once the exit door is closed, so too has that part of a child's life. It is easy to miss some parts of these chapters as they open and close so quickly; the pre-school years and school years are divided into short intervals as the child's life evolves, periods of transition, ever changing. If a parent isn't around to participate in most of these segments in life, then they risk missing important events and milestones that they may later regret and the child gets to clock up absentee parent moments which become filed in their memory bank. Too many missed events will interfere with the formation of a healthy parent-child relationship. Parents can't regain years passed to amend absences and it is often on reflection that they would give anything to be able to. If the parent-child bond is weak or non-existent, relationships are at risk of breaking down. There comes a time in parenthood when you have to put your tools down, step away from the bench and hope that all you have done will be enough. As if it's not, it's too late.

Sometimes ambiguous loss hits hard and, at other times, it presents subtly. In the case of the empty nest syndrome, there is an adjustment period, as a child gathers more and more independence before eventually leaving home completely. As this happens, a grieving process begins which can be likened to a slow breakup of a relationship as it was once known. It's really the same relationship but different. Children do grow into adulthood and it can be difficult to accept the loss of the "child" and all the stages that accompanied that child's growing years. Although love and emotional closeness still holds strong, the tangible, physical closeness gradually dissipates as the relationship takes on a new dimension. The child adapts to this new dimension easily, as the parent has remained constant. The parent, however, has witnessed the child's life unfold, from infancy, through the many stages of childhood, until the emergence of a young adult. Nostalgia often sets in, especially with many reminders: photos, old toys stuffed in cupboards and growth measurements on door frames. There are bound to be periods of mourning and disbelief as the parent reminisces of a life that once was. Throughout this grieving process, it is not uncommon that the parent becomes a little overbearing with paraphernalia of when their child was young. An attempt to reel the child in to revisiting the past may be met with disappointment, when it's realised that the child doesn't share in the same gusto. Instead, the child may only show a mild interest, if at all, partially because their memory is patchy and their experience is so different and partially because they are far more interested in their life as it is in the present tense.

A person can be physically present but psychologically absent, in the occurrence of diminished mental acuity. Brain disease or injury such as acquired brain injury, Parkinson's disease, dementia and Alzheimer's, alter a person's personality and capabilities. Once a normal functioning society member, this person becomes mentally handicapped and, subsequently, suffers a loss of identity, alongside skills they had previously firmly established. As well as dealing with a sense of loss and grief on diagnosis, there often remains an uncertainty surrounding the progression of the condition, adding another layer to the grieving process. Close family members and friends also grieve this loss, complicated by accommodating the new version of their loved one. This altered relationship can conjure up feelings of guilt, frustration, exhaustion and stress. Communication becomes difficult and emotions conflicted as there is no clear understanding of when the loss will be resolved or come to a closure.

Workaholism, alcoholism, drug and substance abuse and mental illness can also cause a psychological absence. This loss can be invisible to others, especially if the affected person still appears to be a functional member of society. Little does anyone know of what transpires behind closed doors and the battle loved ones face in holding together such a turbulent relationship. Time and energy are siphoned from personal relationships into the addiction or illness, causing an emotional disconnection. Antisocial and unpredictable behaviours replace normalcy and there becomes a continuous struggle between hope and despair.

A promised relationship full of hope and security can

disintegrate in separation or divorce. A divergence from the expected. An intimate existence expected to last a lifetime is, instead, replaced with estrangement. Preluding the complete breakdown of such a union, after all attempts are exhausted, to hold onto hope, to the marriage vows or to the sweet resolve of all issues, there may be a challenging period of acceptance. Acceptance of the relationship as is. Unchangeable. The grieving process begins long before the resolve of the relationship. This ambiguous period is a part of the ambiguous loss. Any children of the union will feel a shift in relationships, during which they will feel a loss of what used to be, as they adapt to what is now, in the existing altered family unit. If the relationship was one that involved abuse, then the victim may be rewarded for fleeing the relationship and not receive any condolences for the layer of associated grief attached.

Adoption has several layers of ambiguous loss attached to it. For the adoptee, there is a mystery surrounding the biological family. For the adoptive parents, there is the sorrow surrounding children they were never able to naturally conceive or may have lost through death. For the birth parents, there is the loss of the child or children they placed for adoption. There may be unanswered questions, regrets and a sense of loss that is difficult to resolve. The adoptee and birth parents have to contend with a non-tangible person that resides in the heart but is physically inaccessible.

For those of us with ageing parents, there is a process of letting go of what was and accepting what is. There could be a complete change of roles. The child has become an adult and lost the parent-child relationship once known. The parent, through the ageing process, may revert back to child-like ways and become dependent on the very child he or she once raised.

This reversal of roles usually comes at a time when the offspring are busy with their own families and work commitments, which can add resentment to the equation.

The difficulty with ambiguous loss is that it can complicate and delay the process of grieving and may result in unresolved grief and living in a state of limbo. Unlike regular mourning for something tangibly lost, the grieving process is particularly difficult when closure is non-existent. The only way forward is to accept the loss is real, even though it may not have a time frame.

Feelings of grief, doubt, anger, guilt, depression, isolation, hopelessness and ambivalence can all accompany ambiguous loss. It is all normal. Ambiguous loss happens to all of us in one form or another. The important thing is to accept it is as real a loss as any other. Sometimes these losses can be subtle and you feel they don't warrant getting tied up in knots over. If the emotions listed above relate to you then accept that you may be going through a loss of this nature. Take your time to grieve at your own pace and seek support if you need it.

As difficult as it is to go through grief, however which way it presents, these experiences pave the way for further personal growth. You develop another layer of depth to your being, becoming more compassionate and resilient, which will influence the way you handle future difficult and challenging situations.

DEATH

I was preparing a room for the next admission when I caught Simon in my peripheral vision walking down the corridor.

'Hey Kath.' I looked up. Simon was standing over me.

I hadn't noticed he'd entered the room. Having my full attention, he continued with conviction, 'I'm no longer afraid of death, because I've already entered the light and I tell you Kath, I didn't want to come back from it.'

We had previously spoken about this. Simon had experienced his first brush with death that landed him in a coma. A short while after his profound statement, a rare disease took him back to the light. RIP my beautiful friend.

We live. We die. This, we all know. We speak of our lives, our desires, hopes and dreams for the future, not contemplating that death may take us suddenly. We rarely entertain the thought of death, at least not in our early decades. We know that one day we will die, fall into an eternal sleep, leave the planet, pass over into a different realm, arrive at the pearly gates – yet we know little of what happens after death. Most of us assume we will die when we are old. To die young would be most unfortunate and unfair, so it's best not to entertain the thought.

Not knowing exactly what is beyond this life is somewhat

scary and a subject we talk little about. And so, we concentrate solely on the living part of our existence; death often residing in the far corner of our minds. We are not only apprehensive about our own deaths; we are also concerned about losing our most dear ones through this life transition.

It is easy enough to say goodbye to someone we may never cross paths with again but how do we say goodbye to someone we know, who will soon be departing this life? It's not easy to choose the words. Little, if anything, do we know about their feelings toward impending death, whether they are accepting of the fact or downright petrified. What words can we possibly use to help ease fear, provide comfort, make the dying person feel unafraid, comforted, uplifted? How on earth can we improve the quality of their life by anything we say? Wouldn't it be best to just keep quiet, not face the reality, save the embarrassment of anything inappropriate stumbling out of our mouths? Besides, who knows, a miraculous intervention may occur, God willing, to prolong their life. Our deeply rooted survival instincts program us to fight for our lives, as if we can bypass the inevitable. It feels more comfortable to skirt around the subject of death, discrediting it, to be associated with life.

Death can certainly be an uncomfortable subject. It is far from a popular topic of conversation because society has made it awkward. If it was a more readily discussed subject, perhaps we wouldn't have the same fears and dread of facing immortality. If we know of someone whose curtains are drawing over the stage of their life, few of us will openly bid them farewell with, 'All the best with your death. I hope you transition easily; it's been wonderful having you to share life with.'

We are more likely to keep those thoughts to ourselves

perhaps only voicing them to those who also have close relations to the nearly deceased. We feel more comfortable, although not entirely, with planning a last visit. We mostly try to avoid the subject by talking about mundane issues, being extra careful not to mention anything pertaining to the future and maybe deliver one last bunch of flowers, gesturing the thoughts we find too hard to articulate.

In a century of increasing longevity, we are obsessed with prolonging our lives; we have the option of eating healthier, exercising more and reducing stress. Life expectancy is well into the 80s and 90s now, as opposed to the 50s, as it was in the late 19th century. We live in times of quality health care, advanced technology and medicine. There's almost a false sense of immortality. To take it a step further, a few people around the world have opted to save their bodies to fulfil a dream of immortality.

Cryonics is a method of freezing corpses directly after death. The process occurs within minutes of death, within the first 60 seconds, ideally. Profound hypothermia is created as a way of preserving cellular viability. The body is cooled and injected with chemicals to preserve and prevent ice crystal development in tissues and organs. It is then stored indefinitely in liquid nitrogen, keeping the body in a stable, preserved state until the necessary medical technology arrives, on the premise it ever does, to be able to resurrect the body back to life. Once revived, future science will need to cure the disease that led to death and reverse any damage caused by the freezing process. If this science fiction becomes reality, a second life may be possible. Beyond our scope of comprehension, questions raised include: ethical issues, damage already sustained to tissues and organs through the disease that caused death and the toxic effects of the chemicals used. And would the person that was so meticulously cryogenically preserved really be the same person thawed?

Surviving a serious illness or near-death experience can give someone a different perspective on life. Knowing that life was close to ending, renews an appreciation of the gift of life. All trivialities fly out the window, as priorities take precedence. The important things become crystal clear: spending time with loved ones, clutching onto special moments, fully immersing in the now and giving procrastination a swift kick up the backside. The same applies for those known to be close to demise. There is not a moment to be wasted and life is rediscovered in a similar way as a young child views and experiences everything for the first time.

Unfortunately, it is when we know the end of life is looming that we take the extra effort to appreciate the time we have together. As we don't have a crystal ball, we should always be keeping our connections strong, always, every day, every moment. Life is precious as it is precarious and so we need to live life fully, deepen our connections and let go of trivial matters and regrets.

Time has afforded us the opportunity of choosing to die rather than letting it happen naturally. We are currently in debate on assisted dying. Different countries have different rules regarding euthanasia typically reserved for the terminally ill and many countries but not all, have legalised some form of assisted dying known as Voluntary Assisted Dying (VAD). Depending on the jurisdictions of the country in which we live, we may be able to choose a form of euthanasia as the preferred exit to life. Typically, the general criteria meeting legal requirements are: to be capable of making and communicating health care decisions, to be at least 18 years of age, to be terminally ill with a life expectancy of six months or less and to be a resident of the state in which the law has been passed.

Just as we have a choice to end our lives if we meet the criteria, we can elect to extend our lives. Medical procedures and medications can prolong the inevitable for a few more days, months or even years. Prolonging death beyond its natural duration is now commonplace. Perhaps it is in our difficulty in accepting death that compels us to extend our own life or feel a moral obligation in preserving another's life for as long as possible.

Preventing death is an ongoing scientific phenomenon which equates to medical success. Clinicians are trained in medicine to cure, heal and save and it can be difficult to curb the escalation of treatment, as to do so may be considered negligent or falling short of practising to full scope. Unless otherwise consented, not to resuscitate, all measures will be taken to save a life, whether it be in a clinical setting or at the site of an accident. DNR: Do not resuscitate, is a binding order to not attempt any medical measures to prolong life. Emergency treatment will prevail unless there is a valid written directive to the contrary. Even when the medical team deem it as being futile. If there is not a written order in place, an attempt to actively treat to preserve life will occur irrespective of any circumstances. Not for resuscitation may be a desire that is thought or spoken of, however, if it is not put in writing to become a legal written consent, then resuscitation will be performed, even if it may conflict with a person's condition such as advanced age or terminal illness.

Extensive medical technology can separate the dying from their loved ones in their most vulnerable and final moments. Intimate time spent is often interrupted by medical procedures. Curtains are drawn, families and loved ones are ushered out as procedures are administered to keep death at bay, for that little bit longer. When the curtains open, loved ones may return to the bedside to find the patient further disenabled by the application of more medical apparatus. Speech, facial expression and movement inhibited. In the hope of servicing patients to give them extended time, harsh, aggressive and risky treatments are laid on the table. Some of these treatments will affect quality of life, increase suffering and isolation and, inadvertently, dangle the individual on a cliff's edge, bringing on an earlier than anticipated death. The pursuit of gaining more time becomes a double-edged sword. The hovering question is: when should treatment be applied and when should it be withdrawn? Have there been previous discussions regarding what the patient desires or is it just assumed? Is a less-than-optimal existence, created through medical intervention, better than accepting and enjoying the last stages of existence with a sound mind to recall the fullness of a life already lived? Doctors and patients may misplace their energy on setting all their goals into a cure or prolonged survival, missing opportunities to focus on quality of life left and how best to achieve goals that pertain to end-of-life wishes.

It seems morally right to prolong life and wrong to allow someone an early death before "time". Where do we draw the line? It is commonly assumed we will get to live right through to our most senior years and let's hope that is the case for you and I and all those dear to us. The fact is, people die every day at any age. How as mortal beings, can we decide or predict the time that death should occur? "Too young to die". Sometimes death takes the young and it seems unfair these individuals didn't get to live a full life. Our non-acceptance of a person dying at a young age may very well influence the management of their care or illness. Too young to make their own decisions, regarding treatment and death experience preferences, these individuals are at the mercy of the decisions made by their family/carers. Children with chronic conditions and terminal illness can be subject to the heroics of doing everything possible to delay the inevitable, sometimes interfering with the natural process of death by applying inappropriate life prolonging treatments. The intense grief and unacceptable prognosis of losing a child may meddle with rational thinking and decision making. The disbelief of someone young being sentenced to death is unfathomable. Acceptance of impending death may take time and so, decisions regarding treatments may sway back and forth, as the grieving parent comes to grips with the demise of their dearly beloved child. That child may inadvertently be escalated from hospice to ICU care in attempts to clutch at last straws.

Good intentions to prolong life may instead backfire, causing the patient more pain and suffering than an earlier death may have. All the heroics could very well divide a child from his or her parent in the last stages of the child's life. A child who is in most need of his or her parent cradling them in their arms, holding their hand, showering them with love and reassurance as they pass, instead may be left alone and frightened amongst strangers in a scary, unfamiliar environment, hooked up to machinery. A parent's intention is, of course, to take all measures for the optimal benefit of the child but intense grief may cloud judgement.

Prolonging life by providing intensive treatment can cause unnecessary discomfort. It can prevent measures otherwise taken to allow the departing person one last portion of quality life, however little that may be. Medicalisation of birth is a renowned and accepted practice: manipulating the natural process of birth by bringing life into the world by artificial means. Sometimes necessary. Sometimes not. Death is also medicalised, but is it ever really necessary? Care is escalated to prolong life, bypassing the act of nature. Instead of letting a disease or age take its normal untampered progression, all aides are pulled in an attempt to disguise the truth. That being, the body will, undeniably succumb to death. Medical research and scientific breakthroughs encourage us to believe that cures for illness are within our reach. Even in the most terminal diagnoses. Are we denying dignity to fulfil our own needs of comfort and ignoring the tell-tale signs that death is nigh? Do we even know what those signs are? Are we forfeiting humane care and administering futile treatments because we have lost the ability to accept death and suffering as aspects of our lives?

People hold back on conversations regarding their death. Not only is it a morbid subject but one we believe to be a thing in the distant future that doesn't require our attention just now. So, all too often, it gets left dangling, just hanging there undiscussed. Family members and others close to the dying person have to make calculated decisions according to what they believe their loved one would want. And if they don't know, they may make decisions to fulfil their own desires. While there is still life present, the stance may be taken to do everything possible to save it, especially as there are many new developments and options to do so. If the "talk" isn't had, then the patient may go through undue duress by heroic treatment or unwanted management and miss out on the end of life and death they would have preferred.

Fear and the defences built around death can make it difficult to accept it as a natural progression of life and so, a person with a terminal illness may hold onto a cure, hope of remission or more time. It is in this avoidance of death that comes an unpreparedness, causing us to cling to life, as we only know how to live, not how to die.

If time was dedicated to talking about and making decisions regarding death, then we would be enabled to fulfil a person's wishes rather than having to make the best possible guess for what we may think will suffice for life's inevitable ending. To have knowledge of a person's death wishes, enables us to honour their life in the most respectful and intimate way.

Birth. Our entrance into life is celebrated and plans are made to make it the best possible experience. Birth doulas are sometimes employed to guide us through the delicate birthing process. Just as birth is as intricate as it is delicate, so too is death and there are people trained in assisting both the dying and their loved ones through this transition. Time and consideration are dedicated to formulating a written birth preference document. It empowers the birthing mother to trust and surrender to her birthing instincts. An end-of-life preference document may inspire a new understanding of the dying person or meaning of his or her death. A doula, assisting the death process, can transform the experience from one that is fraught with anxiety, fear and suffering, into one filled with confidence and a sense of sacredness, infused with love.

If a person is aware of their impending death, they can be gently assisted in coming to an acceptance of their fate and in perhaps organising a living wake, whereby the dying person is present and can partake in their own farewell. A doula can aid in the reflection of a life lived and help with constructing written notes, autobiographies and legacies to leave behind. Family members and caregivers are supported and encouraged to take on active roles in the dying process. The padlock on death is unlocked as it becomes accepted as a routine part of existence. This opens opportunities for ceremonies and rituals to be put in place, sharing in desires and preferences concerning the process. Being intimately involved can reduce the associated stress surrounding death and assist in the grieving process that follows. In normal dying, void of any preparation, a family can be waiting on edge for their loved one who is often unconscious, to quietly slip away from the world. Without some sort of plan in place it becomes too late and the bucket list, ceremony or desired ritual isn't achieved.

There may not be any plans put in place for the end, as not all people understand that they have choices. Medical professionals deal with Advance Care Directives, which is a legal document stating a person's preferences in receiving medical care if that person is incapable of making medical decisions. Advance Care Directives guide choices for caregivers and doctors if a person is incapacitated to do so through serious injury, illness or dementia. Also known as a living will. If there is no legal documentation in place, everything will be done to preserve life, including resuscitation when the heart ceases to pump and breathing has stopped. Doulas and other chosen support people can be involved in planning a living will incorporating choices regarding the desired place of death, the arrangement of the room congruent with end of life wishes, writing letters/a journal, help with composing an obituary, help with sorting affairs and unfinished business and assistance in deciding who, if anyone, will be present during the death transition.

Too often, people are dying alone as death and dying have become more and more medicalised with advancing technology. One last attempt to prolong life trumps letting a patient succumb to the inevitable and the sacredness of death is stolen. Wouldn't it feel better to die in an environment conducive to death? Holding a loving hand, enveloped in someone's arms, being supported and feeling loved throughout the process? The room infused with soft music and aromatherapy, curtains open to let in the warm sunshine or closed to create a soft ambience. To have people surrounding you that are accepting of your passage, whispering comforting words, gently leading you into the light/passage/afterlife. How different would it feel to be in a cold clinical setting? Alone? Loved ones refusing to let you go, not accepting, begging you to stay alive or not being able to face being with you during your transition?

In western society, it is commonplace that a person will die in a hospital or hospice. Or even in the back of an ambulance or in an emergency department. Sometimes this simply can't be helped but there are times when other choices can be made.

Few people are given the dignity of dying at home because relatives/loved ones are ill equipped to provide palliative care. We are generally unfamiliar with what to do, how to cope. It is more likely, however, that a person dying at home will be surrounded by loved ones during their demise. In a hospital setting, even when relatives are called in, there is a risk of not getting there in time or missing the event by stepping outside during a procedure or to take a short break. Or it could simply be a case of miscommunication.

When my father died, my mother and I had left the hospital the night before knowing he was in a stable condition yet leaving instructions for the staff to call us if there was any sign of deterioration. We were notified early that morning some hours after his death. When someone misses their loved one's passing, there is a certain amount of guilt accompanying the grief. If only I had stayed. Why weren't my instructions clearer? Was there something else going on in the ward at the time preventing the staff from making the call and, if so, was he inadvertently neglected? How did he feel alone? Was he scared?

On our return to the hospital that morning, we said our goodbyes, regretting that even in death he had lain there alone for a few hours before we arrived. A few hours before we were even contacted. I knew the protocol that followed. The hospital staff had been patient in waiting for the family to attend but they needed to transfer him to the morgue as they required the ward bed. My father died of lung cancer. He had decided not to go down the path of chemo. Dad had gone into hospital for a short stint and was doing well. He was to have some tests and then be discharged home the following day. A chest infection complicated matters and he succumbed to his disease. Before his rapid decline, it seemed he was powering through this terminal illness, giving us a glimmer of false hope.

Two years beforehand, as he was waiting for his diagnostic chest x-ray, he turned to the nurse of the family and said, 'If this is cancer, do you think I will get about two years?'

I didn't know how to answer him in a non-clinical way. I was factual and never really discussed his illness with him. Apart from knowing his preference to forgo chemotherapy, to keep some quality of life while he still had it, I had no idea on how he preferred to die. And like many others who later reflect on their loved one's death, I have regrets. I pushed the subject aside so as to go about living as normal, throwing a blanket over reality. Why didn't I talk about it with him? I simply really didn't know how. But I so now wish I did.

Should a person know that they are dying? Grave news can come as a shock but when delivered with empathy and compassion it can enable the dying person to feel supported and better equipped to work through the accompanying rollercoaster of emotions. Knowing allows a person to physically and emotionally prepare for their death. It allows them a choice on how they want to spend the rest of their time and who they would like to spend their time with. It gives them time to put plans in place, deal with unfinished business and to strengthen or mend relationships.

Avoidance of the truth robs a person's chance of spending the rest of their life in the way that they want to. Emotions go unexpressed and wishes unfulfilled as conversations are avoided. Interactions may become superficial in an effort to keep up the pretence. Fear, isolation and depression may set in as the dying person has no one available to talk to or share their concerns with. They may feel alone and become withdrawn, unable to derive any pleasure from life's moments. Understandably, part of the reason the truth may be withheld from the dying person is in the hope that the person can still withdraw pleasure from life, rather than falling into a state of depression. Yet withholding the truth can deny the person reflection, leading to inner healing and have a profound effect on relationships. It can also deny loved ones the opportunity to share their most heartfelt feelings and to truly engage in life lived fully. Secrecy and misinformation can cause false hope and eventual resentment. Intuitively, the dying may be well aware of their fate but feel displaced from life by those around them who want to protect them. The act of dying then becomes lonely and impersonal and the suffering can become far greater than the physical illness itself. Feeling disempowered and disconnected from their loved ones, the dying may quietly slip away alone and unnoticed.

A dying person need not be considered as "diseased". They need to be treated as the person that they are: living in the moment as we all are, open to the joys and gifts of life as they present themselves, with permission to live their life as a dying person and permission to die uninhibited when the time presents.

The majority of people still die in hospital beds or hospices, sometimes still attached to monitors or noisy machinery. These are the expected places to be taken for death to occur or, maybe for an attempt to prolong life or, purely because society is hugely unequipped to deal with death outside these institutions, if given a choice. Wouldn't it be better, where possible, to die at home surrounded by familiar sights, scents, sounds and those most dear to you? Of course, death can take you suddenly and you may not get a choice. Not all plans made, may come to fruition; wishes may change or you may be dying before you become consciously aware of it. Having planned death preferences still allows the living to honour your existence and cushion the grieving process that follows your demise.

Definition of a "good death" is different for everybody. Perhaps it is a death in sleep or a death following everything that could have been done, was. Or perhaps, a death following a fulfilling life or one that occurred in an environment where the last hours were encompassed by peace and love. Not everyone would necessarily prefer to die at home or in a hospice. For some a hospital may be the preferred setting. Once a person's dead we can't then ask them how they rated their death.

Choices matter in death, just as they do in life. Some people may prefer to die within the presence of family and friends sitting close to them at the bedside or even being caressed by a loved one or having that loved one share the bed to be held, comforting them as they pass over. Others may prefer to die alone or eliminate the amount of closeness to others, as it may interfere with the internal process of dying, pulling them back into involvement in a world they are in the process of leaving.

As a young nurse, I was often witness to the dying. On the second day of my ward orientation, I was sent into a curtained cubicle to lay out a newly deceased patient. Without pre-warning or counselling, my instructions were to wash the patient, tag him and make sure to put his false teeth back in his mouth, which I was told was the most challenging part of the procedure. Suddenly, there I was, peering over an ashen corpse that I had to somehow prepare for the morgue. A pair of yellow dentures sat in a silver mug. A bowl of soapy water, sheets, tags and labels were positioned on the bedside table. As I lifted his limbs, it dawned on me, the meaning of "dead weight". Awkward. Heavy. It was like I was lifting a brick or sack of sand. Although the curtains confined us together, we couldn't be more separate. Two bodies, each in the same vicinity but in separate realms. My only previous experience with death was that of a dead uncle whom, dressed in a suit, laid neatly in an open coffin, my brother dared me to view as a child. For the first time, I was confronted with a "patient" of the same nature. However, this person was freshly dead, naked and not at all cosmetically presentable as my embalmed uncle had been. A real-life dead human. Now a corpse. Still, waxlike, no longer breathing with hard rubber jaws I could not mould those wretched teeth around. Behind the curtains, I stood alone with a man whose discharge from hospital would be as a cadaver via the mortuary. In those few moments, which felt like an eternity, I thought about my nursing career and all that lay ahead and vowed that the best way through the inevitable, was to become detached from the rawness of death.

As the months rolled forward, I experienced more death. It was something I preferred to avoid. In nursing school, we didn't have any training on how to manage death or death's grieving loved ones and so, we fumbled through it the best way we could. We learned the basics of laying out a body. The nitty gritty part of dealing with a person dying. The more personal aspects of death and dying were left up to the medical staff as they were more apt at explanations based on their medical knowledge. They too, were inept as their training didn't include a holistic approach. It was only through experience and maturity that these skills would develop and so the senior staff were better at it.

Apart from keeping the dying as comfortable as possible, I was unprepared on how to assist them mentally or spiritually. It was a blessing for me if someone had passed during my tea break, as I could then avoid the awkwardness of not knowing how to handle death, what to say or how best to comfort them in their last moments. On my return, my job would be to lay out the patient, and then transfer him or her to the morgue. This, I became well equipped to do. Once a patient commenced the tell-tale rattle of Cheyne-Stokes breathing, my aim would be to scurry off quickly, hoping the half hour tea break would be time enough to miss the final breath.

I remember once, when being on a stint of night shift, one of the patients in the medical ward wouldn't settle. After the late evening tidy round of placing bedside chairs in corridors, Mrs Insomniac would demand to remain sitting in hers and would insistently cry out, 'Come here nurse, I'm dying!'

This would go on for a couple of hours until she fell asleep upright in her chair, night after night. Eventually, we would get her into bed and by morning, she would be fine, until nightfall, when the same behaviour would resume. After attending to her several times, she would quieten, only for a few minutes before the crescendo started over. I assumed she was senile, just demanding attention, so I ignored her pleas, until one night there was silence. Sometimes death comes unexpectedly.

In the prime of my youth, death was abstract, even though I was witness to serious illness and death. During my second-year placement in theatre, a surgeon once called upon his students to step up closer to the operating table, so we could get a better view of what lay beneath the thoracotomy he had just performed on a middle-aged man. There, in the chest cavity, lay a pair of black organs. It was a vast contrast to the pinkness of the surrounding tissue.

'Now girls, this is how your lungs look if you smoke and this man is only a light smoker,' he explained as he cupped his hand around one of the diseased lungs.

As shocking as it was, it didn't deter me from lighting up a cigarette a few hours later and to continue my habitual addiction for many years to follow. I was young, I was invincible, at least for a good while yet. These were my thoughts. It was easy to dismiss the reality of disease and the associated consequences when death was far from my present realm. Or so I believed.

Hospitals signify sickness and death. You go to hospital if you need an operation or treatment for an illness. Usually, you are discharged when you are well enough, although some people never get to leave. It may be assumed that a hospital setting is the best place for a person who is gravely ill. There are certain support structures set up for the dying and their loved ones, however, they can sometimes be minimised due to shift schedules, the number of patients they are required to serve, as well as after hours and weekend limitations. Not to mention staff shortages. With reduced resources, there are times when the family and close support people are left to deal with the situation in the best way possible, sometimes leaving them to feel abandoned, alone and ill prepared.

Feelings and conversations that were meant to be shared before death sometimes aren't, as we don't want to bring up a morbid subject or become depressed thinking about the loss of someone close. In the case of someone suffering a terminal illness, there may be a death plan prepared. In this instance, it is more likely that conversations have already been broached regarding death, than it is if death comes early or is sudden. On reflection, there can be a lot of regret regarding subjects not discussed and a feeling of guilt for not having the guts to talk about a sensitive subject following the demise of someone close. Did they have the funeral/burial they would have wanted? Did they feel truly loved and cherished before they left us? Did we give them the attention they deserved or were we too caught up in our own lives? What were their desires and wishes? Were these kept hidden because it wasn't a thing to talk about?

Because of the ability to hold back death, it's easy to deny the inevitability of life ending. The mentality of death not being associated with life, keeps it comfortably suppressed. We talk of birth, of living, but not so much of death. And because this topic is skimmed over, if at all ever discussed, we revoke a person's, as well as our own, rite of passage from one realm to another.

People may harbour guilt because they missed the death, didn't take time to discuss the dead person's wishes, didn't spend more time with them before the death, didn't say sorry, heal an emotional wound, didn't say 'I love you', 'thank you', didn't touch, hug, kiss or hold their hand. That death occurred in a hospital when the wish was for it to occur at home. That medical intervention possibly took away dignity, comfort, diminished the opportunity of reflection and propped up a barrier isolating the dying person from their loved ones.

Dying in the presence of a loved one can provide a sense of deep comfort if the support given is unhindered by reservations. Unfortunately, not knowing how to act/cope with impending death can cause a dying person to pass away feeling disconnected to their loved ones. Denial and extreme grief can be so overpowering it can create a wedge between the loved one and the dying at the very time they need closeness. When death occurs, those left behind can face tremendous guilt because of this, impacting the grieving process.

Some people are plucked from life's game before the finish line. That is, what we assume the finish line should be: eighth, ninth, 10th decade. I have worked in the same hospital now for 30 years. Throughout that period, a handful of colleagues I had shared my breaks with in the common tearoom, have since been intermittently erected as obituary photos on the noticeboard that sits directly across from the tearoom table. It seems incredulous that the people I once conversed and laughed with over a cup of coffee, later shared the same space as memorial pictures on a pin board. Disease and tragedy had taken these select few prior to their senior years. One of them had been a student I mentored and another was one of my dearest friends. Even though my beautiful friend left this world suddenly, we shared conversations about death and the afterlife as we believed it to be. The grieving process was softened by knowing his beliefs and carrying out his wishes.

Talk about death. It's difficult. It's sad. But it's inevitable. The better we prepare, the easier it is for those left behind. Live your days and put some plans in place for the type of death you want, if it ends up you have a choice. Death may take you by surprise, so it is good to decide now on how you would like to be remembered: legacy, rituals and what type of memorial/funeral service you would like. In the scheme of things, life spans out over just a few decades, nine to 10 at most. Spend quality time with those important to you, make your mark on the world, achieve your innermost desires, create art, get on with the project you have been procrastinating about, don't hold onto grudges, mend broken relationships where possible, and prioritise. Technology may have the ability to prolong life but no matter what, we cannot choose life over death.

Death is shattering. It seems our whole world stops the moment a loved one passes and yet all around us, it is still in motion. How can people continue to act normally when one of them has suddenly exited the planet? Death is mysterious. There is a disbelief coupled with wonder when life comes to an end. It is the ultimate magic trick and amidst the grief that follows death, there is a sliver of envy that the mystery of death is revealed to those who pass through the veil of life. Eventually, the life game will conclude for each and every one of us and it is only natural to be afraid of the end as we will enter unknown territory.

Who knows, we could be in a life reincarnated in which case we have already experienced death and just have no memory of it. Can any of us think back to what or where we were before conception? There was a time before we had any conceived memories. That didn't seem like a scary time. In a previous world of reduced life span, when war, famine, slavery and childhood mortality were prevalent, suffering was intensified and so death was looked upon as a release from this world to a better life. Perhaps we fear death more in western cultures as life expectancy has increased and the less it's openly discussed, the scarier it becomes. Fear of the unknown is a universal part of humanity, whatever your beliefs are. Trust in the universe. It has it all worked out. We shall go with the flow, as those before us already have.

CONCLUSION

Informally enrolled in the school of life here on planet earth, our lessons begin from the moment of our arrival and continue until the end of our existence. In the beginning of life, we are highly dependent on other human beings for our survival, which slowly tapers off as we evolve and mature. Our destination, our human guides and the availability of resources, will all have a bearing on how we begin our life journey.

We all have separate lives with so many similarities and similar lives with so many differences. Although our lives are different, we share the same human emotions and so, we can relate to one another on many levels. This is the reason we fare better in life when we play it alongside others. People come in and out of our lives bearing gifts of love, companionship, generosity, diversity and wisdom. We make connections to many human equivalents and despite these connections being transient or permanent, they are all instrumental in our evolution as human beings.

In early infancy, we begin to establish a consciousness which is very basic and immature. From a sensory awareness of body, self, and the world, our self-awareness gradually expands to become more complex and, as we gain experiences, we begin to lay down the many layers that constitute our internal programming. All our conditioning, influenced by our thoughts and belief patterns, is stored in the subconscious mind which drives our behaviour. As our awareness and sense of self matures, we recognise that society expects us to behave in a certain way and so we customise our behaviour to socially acceptable standards. We conform to what's expected of us, sometimes keeping our true feelings hidden. But the mask we wear doesn't always conceal the truth, as we communicate in a very sophisticated way. Body language is astute in revealing the sincerity behind verbal communication and once we grasp its power, the better equipped we are to understand the nuts and bolts behind human behaviour.

Technology has unequivocally simplified and complicated our lifestyles. It has transformed communication and skewed circadian rhythms. Multifunctional skills are required to exist in our presently combined real and digital worlds. Technology has certainly revolutionised the medical field and consequently extended our human lifespan. Definitely a wonderful achievement, however, this lengthened life expectancy may have caused us to shy away from the inevitable part of life, which is death. Technology has enhanced our connections, which has freed barriers of communication. It has also opened up a whole arena of information and entertainment. We must learn to incorporate these advantages into our world in a healthy manner. Otherwise, the addictive nature of personalised technology can cultivate a preoccupation in digital worlds, with a disconnect to intuition and an increased attentiveness to what others have that we don't. Mind respite is less on the agenda than it once was and we tend to get edgy if we have nothing to do to fill in our time. Unaccustomed to this nothingness, it becomes more difficult to draw our attention away from the callings of our digital devices. Any vacancies can be filled and we have to make a concerted effort to give the mind back what it deserves; total reprieve.

As a human race we make observations of others sharing our planet and discover (or sometimes just make the assumption – because maybe it's just an illusion) that there are some people better off and some people worse off than ourselves. In our pursuit to improve our current status in life, we are more inclined to focus on those who are richer, more popular, better looking or more successful and we strive for ways to achieve similar results. This can motivate us to be the best version of ourselves but we must be careful not to be judgemental or allow self-doubt to dismiss our already established unique attributes and accomplishments.

Our expectations in life aren't always met and so we have to adapt and board an alternate life carriage. This can be difficult and we may swear and curse at the unfairness of it all. Life can suddenly become a bit or, a lot, harder and we need to pull out all stops to rebalance and create a desirable way forward. On reflection, it is often the hurdles we face in life that build on our resilience and empowerment. It's all about making the best choices with the hand of cards we have. Adversity and life changing events delve deep into our pocket of resources, transforming our lives in one way or another. Definitely for the better, if we apply the value from the lesson. A less than ideal hand can still come up trumps if the cards are played right.

The story of our life comprises of past, present and future, which are all intertwined in our measure of happiness. Our recollections of the past aren't always accurate and we cannot foresee into the future, only imagine it. And yet, our thoughts spend far too much time wallowing in what was and what might be, ignoring what is. The present is the most precious time we have. It is what we do with our now that will have a bearing on our past and future. To access the grandeur of now, involves unleashing fear, regret and worry; emotions that bubble up from a blabbering mind, distracting us from real-life as it is presently playing.

Time is our constant companion until it's not. Our personal time here on earth is unknown but as sure as we are mortal, one day, we'll have none left. Not only is it important to decide how we want to spend our time, it is as equally imperative to consider how much of it, if any, we are prepared to waste. Making time a priority in life counts right now, as you can never be certain of your tomorrows. Be honest with your time, set some boundaries and don't be deluded by time leeches. Deception can easily steal your most prized possession.

We all create our own life stories and like reading a good book we want our chapters to reflect a life well lived. Throughout the narrative of our life, we choose how we want to construct our chapters. Our choices will have a tremendous influence on our health, prosperity and happiness. Some of our past chapters may reveal components of our lives that we wish we could have shaped differently. All our chapters, desired or otherwise, are instrumental in our life lessons. Rather than have regrets, we can learn from our experiences and we can reset our life story by applying our values, principles and wisdom. As long as we are still in the game, we have new chapters to write and we can proceed with these enthusiastically, knowing they will be all the more embellished.

It's difficult to deal with and talk about the serious issues in life. But we all must go through them, so it's important to have some knowledge that may resonate and hopefully lighten the burden of the hardships we face. When life gets tough, support is paramount and as many hands lighten the load, they can also build a bridge of strength.

Wherever you are in your life journey, each phase comes with obstacles and challenges leading you to the next destination. As one chapter folds, there'll always be another that opens. Always. Including the time when we transition from this earthly realm.

www.ingramcontent.com/pod-product-compliance
Lightning Source LLC
Chambersburg PA
CBHW030547080526
44585CB00012B/292